AMERICAN BREAD

CHRONIC LYME DISEASE AND THE TAO OF THE OPEN ROAD

AMERICAN BREAD

CHRONIC LYME DISEASE AND THE
TAO OF THE OPEN ROAD

NICK VITTAS

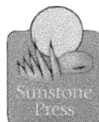

Sunstone
Press

SANTA FE

The names of many of the characters in this book have been changed,
though the events and places are factual.

Sunstone books may be purchased for educational, business, or sales promotional use.
For information please write: Special Markets Department, Sunstone Press,
P.O. Box 2321, Santa Fe, New Mexico 87504-2321.

Book and Cover design › Vicki Ahl
Body typeface › Calibri
Printed on acid-free paper
∞

Library of Congress Cataloging-in-Publication Data

Vittas, Nick, 1977-
   American bread : chronic Lyme disease and the tao of the open road / by Nick Vittas.
      pages cm
   ISBN 978-0-86534-903-2 (softcover : alk. paper)
   1. Vittas, Nick, 1977---Health. 2. Lyme disease--Patients--United States--Biography.
3. Chronic diseases--Patients--United States--Biography. I. Title.
   RC155.5.V58 2012
   616.9'2460092--dc23
   [B]
                                        2012029172

WWW.SUNSTONEPRESS.COM
SUNSTONE PRESS / POST OFFICE BOX 2321 / SANTA FE, NM 87504-2321 /USA
(505) 988-4418 / ORDERS ONLY (800) 243-5644 / FAX (505) 988-1025

To my Mom and Dad,
thank you for all your love and support.

Preface

When I was laid up sick I read Jack Kerouac's *On the Road* and my heart salivated for the chance to sweep over the country in the bold, wild brush strokes of a mad, continental painter. *Dharma Bums* elevated the Sierra Nevadas into a mythical wonderland in my eyes and, after reading Ken Kesey's *One Flew Over the Cuckoo's Nest,* my little soul ached to rush with McMurphy through the great northwest. But I was stuck in DC. Book after book passed through my reading stand (my hands were unable to hold a book) and the adventures therein began to symbolize more than just a trek across a row of States to me. I saw freedom in the endless stream of highways to choose from. I saw adrenaline in the wild, foreign landscapes and bevy of changing faces and cities. I saw vitality and endurance in hurling oneself into the unknown. In short, I saw the opposite of sickness. But as my health corroded my world slowly shrank into smaller and smaller circles. First I became confined to the DC area, then to my house, and then nearly to my bed itself, and with each diminishing circle the longing urge to break free and fly down the road heading west grew stronger, into an insatiable craving, my own version of the American dream.

I wouldn't fully entertain that wanderlust within me because to do so felt fruitless. Nothing could have been further from my reality than to pack into a shit-box car and go. I just knew that if I ever got a chance to live that dream, I would feast on it. Often when people are denied something for long enough, the need molds itself upon their psyche, and this imprint prods them along even after the dire time of deprivation has long passed. I saw this phenomenon in my grandparents who grew up in the food shortages that Greece experienced during the Second World War. In those days scarcity of food was a fact. There was no guarantee of a meal the next day, so when they had one, they ate it voraciously. Not a single scrap was spared. Even long after the war, wasting food was viewed as the ultimate sin. My grandfather would eat rotten meat, knowing full well that he'd be sick the next day, simply because the compulsion to eat was ingrained in him. To this day eating is a measure of a man's character to Greeks. Clearing your plate is not your goal; it is your duty. That mentality from the wartime scarcity has been passed on through generations. And so it was with my appetite for the road. It was a blind hunger.

I wanted my own slice of American Bread. I yearned to breathe the crisp air of the Rockies, to see them grow as I raced across the Colorado plains. I'd never seen a big sky before, not like the sky that stretches out across Montana, and I lavished the idea of standing miniscule before it. I wanted to see the neon madness of Vegas and the rolling uniformity of the flatlands. I longed to hear the blues of Chicago, Memphis, Nashville, Austin, and the swinging Jazz of the Big Easy. Woody Guthrie and Johnny Cash songs revered the sacred beauty of places far away and mysterious to me, like the Redwoods, Mexico, and Arizona, and I craved to touch them all. California has been a national obsession since the gold rush of the 1800s, and as the State's own unique culture evolved it permeated into countless folk and blues songs. I heard them all, and they spoke to me. Texas has a larger than life brand upon it as well. Lightin' Hopkins is guilty of lamenting over both states, and the way he and countless other blues sages mourned landmarks and cities all across the country spurred my curiosity to break the bread of the land and gorge my spirit on its nectar.

In John Steinbeck's *Travels with Charley* he says that Americans are a traveling breed of people, that their ancestors were the ones who pursued the great unknown across the Atlantic, that these rootless wanderers were driven by some compulsion to gamble on a new life, on a new land. Perhaps their ancestors passed on the restless gene and all Americans are bound to ramble, or at least be intrigued by it. To this day the cross-country trip is an American tradition, a rite of passage. I wasn't even born here, but once I got here, it didn't take me long to figure that the American adventure lay behind a steering wheel and an open highway. This realization probably has roots all the way back to the frontier, but you can see it in all forms of American myth and media today.

And when I finally got well enough to pack up and embark, I discovered for myself that the treasures of the road are innumerable and free, and, best of all, unexpected. I wondered if the spirit of all travelers kept gems like eating a sandwich on a cliff along California Highway 1, or a five dollar blues show at T.C.'s lounge on Austin's eastside, hidden in his pocket, tossing them out to those that have the foresight to play it loose, because loose is the only way to play it with the array of choices a road trip continually offers.

American Bread is the best of America. It's far from the money obsessions and consumerism that plague our culture and paint it in a shallow light. American Bread is the beautiful sounds that one's pain can morph into with a guitar, a harmonica, and 12 bars. American Bread is the spontaneous wanderlust that can carry one clear across the continent on a system of highways that trace over a map like veins on a leaf. American Bread is the soul of folk and jazz and country. We invented all those sounds and they sprang from the land like seeds watered with heartache and joy, and everything in between. American Bread is the restless maniac in all of us who craves to get up and go because he's only at peace when he's moving. American Bread is barreling down the road with no plan and nothing on your mind but the rolling backdrop and an overwhelming sense of freedom.

Lessons of Lyme

Like a seasoned poker player who only remembers his coolers and bad beats, along with a handful of monster pots he's won, while everything else fades into a blur, I only remember landmarks, both up and down, along my journey with Lyme disease. I remember the first time I felt a pop in the side of my head, as I was banging out a set of push-ups, way back in December of 1997, and the brutal headaches that followed. Two weeks later I was looking down at a rack of CDs and realized that I couldn't tilt my head slightly downward without the muscles in my neck seizing into spasm. I remember the first time the pain spread from my head and neck to the rest of my body in the summer of 1998. It was twinge in my back as I was riding a bike high on several bong hits, still heavily in denial that I was sick. Of course that realization started to be harder to block when my back stayed locked in pain and stiffness for another three years. The day my hands shot numb from merely holding a book rattled me, and I began to fear that there was no end to what I could lose. And when the pain spread to my legs in the summer of 2000 I nearly gave up. That was when the disease knocked me on my back.

I remember the first time I was happy again, in the fall of 2000, a month before my eventual diagnosis. I was walking up a hill in a thunderstorm when it all clicked for me. I remember how shocked I was when I got the phone call from the doctor giving me a diagnosis and a course of action and slowly seeing improvements in my body as months, and years, of antibiotic treatments moved on. The first time I wore a backpack with a book and several videos in it, and didn't feel as if the bag was filled with boulders, stands out as the first time I knew the antibiotics were forcing the disease to retreat. I was waiting in a subway tunnel with a sly grin as the train pulled up. Soon after I held a book in my hands, tentative at first, only trying to grasp it while lying down, so my elbows could rest against the bed, then all bold and sitting up. I remember the first time I played basketball again, awkward and out of sync from a five-year hiatus, but bounding around the court with enthusiasm because I knew it was a gift. When I finally built the strength to put a set of 45-pound plates on the bench press I felt I'd truly arrived, and there was no turning back. That was in the spring of 2003.

A couple of years later, in the spring of 2005, I got cocky and pushed my body too hard, playing basketball four or five times a week over the course of six months. I recall sitting on the couch, watching TV as my legs started hurting again, and knowing that it would be years before they stopped. By 2007 my body had come back strong. I had the good fortune to fall into a teacher's aide position in a local preschool, and thus enjoyed a series of wild trips around the continent during the summers of 2006 and 2007.

As 2008 arrived I took the confidence gained from these trips and geared to step back on the basketball court. But it was not to be. I sprained my back in February of that year and knew, with the same sickening instinct, that I'd be in pain for a long time. I reluctantly abandoned all workouts except for swimming then. Around April of 2009 I swam a little too hard, rushing through a set of laps despite the fact that I could feel the back of my head getting tighter and tighter. I just wanted to swim and ignored the warning signal. The next day I had a headache that was so deeply rooted in the thin muscles coating my skull that I knew that the pain was there to stay, that I'd fallen and would have to start over again.

But there's more to it than just these mileposts recording my physical condition over a fourteen year run with a chronic disease that just won't quit. There's a whole separate timeline, a whole other set of landmarks that are harder to spot out individually because they blend into the background of my body's progressions and regressions. This hidden timeline is defined by shifts in my character, instances when Lyme disease forced me to evolve. Throughout the past fourteen years the disease has demanded that I change specific patterns of thought, adopt new philosophies, mine within my experiences for adaptations to my behaviors. Often the only alternative the disease offered me was to suffer in misery. And so I changed. I evolved at the hand of the disease.

Sometimes these evolutions can be pinpointed to a specific date, the first time I meditated, the month I picked up a guitar, and other times they kind of grew in the shadows of necessity, taking form gradually, with no real beginning or end. The discipline to stay sober, and the realization that happiness is best served by flexibility both fall into the latter category.

Many of these lessons directly correlate to the road, for it seems that not only did my experiences with Lyme disease drive me out onto the road, but they also prepared me for it too. The equanimity I developed in the course of dealing with chronic illness proved to be the perfect running mate for all the unpredictable turns a road trip can take.

So much of who I am today has been spurred into creation by a disease that

I've been actively trying to rid myself of for the past fourteen years. It's a strange juxtaposition. That being said, I won't ever give up on being fully healthy. Lyme taught me that as well.

Missing In Action
June 23–June 27, 2007

> "Because they [sages] do not contend,
> the world can not contend with them."
> —Lao Tzu

I had a brutal night of cards at the casinos off Lake Tahoe's south shore. The kind of night that makes me curse my greedy heart for leading me back to the poker tables in pursuit of that crackling feeling that sweeps over me when I've just won money. I sullenly walked back to our hotel room disgusted with myself and wondered when I would retire the gamble for good. I fell asleep with a bitter film over my thoughts only to wake up in the early morning hours with the remnants of a dream flickering in my mind like a worn out movie projector that can only show a handful of frames at a time. I started to piece the dream together as I took a leak. In the dream two thugs had stolen my beloved Honda. I had been in a city and stupidly left the keys in the ignition and these kids had sped off with my car when I had turned my back, laughing at all the stuff they were going to pawn. I sped after them on foot, and through some surreal blend of will and fantasy that seems so natural in dreams, I managed to regain possession of my car. Costa roused as I returned to my bed and I told him about the dream. "What? Go check on her," Costa demanded. He had taken to calling the car "her" like I did. He had only been on the road with her for a week, but already a love for her was creeping its way into his speech. She's a wonderful car, so it's only natural.

"Honda, protect yourself," I called out to her and flopped back onto the bed.

Costa and I had left a week earlier from DC. I was slated to spend the whole summer on the road, while Costa would accompany me for the first three weeks. Costa Demas is a friend of mine I've known since tenth grade, over 13 years at that point. He is half Greek and half Peruvian, on the short and stocky side, but somehow always surrounded by a girl or two. He's got a charming cleft chin that all the girls swoon over, and those dark, deeply set eyes, which so many Greeks seem to have. Our chosen mode of transportation was my 1996 black Honda Accord. The car was battle tested, churning out 17,000 miles on a series of cross-country trips the previous summer without so much as a hiccup. You roll like that with a car and she finds a space in your heart right quick.

California highway 50 was our route through the Sierra Nevadas and into the Bay area. It's a simple, two-lane strip of pavement deftly carved into the mountains, perfect for a meditative ride that energizes something basic in the core of a man. Within hours we were idling in traffic, waiting to cross the Bay Bridge. I'd been applying pressure on Costa to forgo the Bay area and shoot north in order to enjoy the adventures that awaited us in Oregon and beyond. But I deferred to Costa as to whether he would relent to the social squeeze his uncle's high school buddy was laying on him to come visit him in Oakland. To see Costa's uncle's buddy we had to spend one more night in Tahoe, then a night in Oakland, then finally proceed to Oregon. It's all very complicated, I know, so you can imagine how I felt trying to weed some sense out of what happened. That extra night in Tahoe turned my profit of 275 dollars in our first night of gambling to a net loss of 75 after I lost 350 during our extra night at Tahoe's casinos. I agreed to go visit Costa's uncle's buddy in hope that if we got some of the social bullshit that inevitably comes with going anywhere with Costa out of the way early, I would have a license to skip all the other acquaintances Costa had blabbered our plans to and now felt obligated to visit in Portland and God knows where else.

Costa called his uncle's high school buddy, who went by the nickname Tubby. Tubby had a place out in Oakland and Costa had agreed to go spend one night with him and then leave at the crack of dawn for Oregon. There was no answer. We slowly crept to the tollbooth, and having heard nothing from this man, crossed the bridge and found our way into San Francisco's Chinatown for a late lunch.

Tubby had been pressuring Costa to go to, of all things, a Goo Goo Dolls concert for the last couple of days. At my strong insistence Costa had tried to find some socially responsible way out of the visit, but to no avail. Costa called him and left a voicemail. We still didn't have the guy's address and as the clock inched toward six, I became optimistic that we might escape Oakland altogether, stay in San Fran for dinner, then shoot north toward Oregon in the night. Costa's phone rang right as I became convinced Tubby was going to let us slip through his fingers. Tubby was on the line, strong arming Costa to visit him in Oakland as I waived my arms in protest, mouthing "No" repeatedly as Costa gave up ground and finally relented to turn back around and meet in Oakland as soon as possible. "What the hell did you do that for," I moaned, agitated that we hadn't found a way out of this snare.

"You don't understand," Costa, pleaded. "He's so persistent, he wouldn't fucking quit. He was all 'come on, I got these girls over, come on, you're gonna have a great time. I already bought your ticket, but you gotta hurry.' I couldn't say no, Nick."

"No," I screamed to show him how easy it is to say. "No," I said it again.

"Come on Nick," Costa said disheartened, with big, round, sad eyes that pleaded for some understanding. "I'm on vacation."

"All right malaka," I grumbled. Malaka means jerk off in Greek, and basically ends almost every sentence between men in the motherland. And so we, just a couple of malakes, found ourselves heading back over the bridge, east toward Oakland, to stay with this guy Tubby for one night.

I pulled the trusty Honda, valiant steed of all my travels across the continent so far, up to Tubby's place on Vernon Street. The neighborhood looked decent enough, resembling more of a middle class feel than the crime den I'd heard Oakland was. Tubby opened the door and I immediately saw that he wasn't fat at all, he was actually in pretty decent shape for a 46 year old. He had a rigid, square jaw line and an only slightly less square head. His small, brown, beady eyes peered out at the world, somehow able to simultaneously radiate dullness while jumping to and fro like a live wire. An overly enthusiastic grin never left Tubby's square face and he bounced everywhere he went, as if there was some mechanism inside him that forced him to bob up and down while moving in any direction. He was also definitely balding and definitely pretending not to be, taking what little hair time had left him on the front of his head, growing it extra long, then combing and gelling it into the right places so that someone who was incredibly near sighted might have the impression that he wasn't losing his hair. He wore tight jeans and an even tighter shirt, and walked around (bobbed really) with his arms bent at the elbows, his lower back arched and his shoulders hunched forward like he was ready to start flexing at the drop of a dime. He was also spectacularly bow legged, to the point that when he walked he gave the impression that he'd forgotten to wipe his ass and was trying to keep his butt cheeks as far away from each other as possible.

His house was nice in an old, quirky kind of way. There were a bunch of curiously eccentric features throughout the place, like a tiny closet sized room with a toilet in it and a slightly larger room with a bathtub and sink directly next to it, or the fact that none of the cupboards had doors in the kitchen. The entire layout of the house seemed to be randomly decided upon, almost like it was put together with the left over scraps of several other houses. Tubby bounced around with a confident bravado that was betrayed by his nervousness. "I like this house," I told him. "It has a lot of character."

"It has a lot of character," Tubby repeated, laughing emphatically as he slapped my back. He was always laughing at inappropriate comments like "my drinking days are over" or "Costa likes to sleep late." These mild, neutral comments would set him off on a round of boisterous, horribly forced laughter that was usually followed by a playful punch or the exhausting demand that we dap it up fist to fist. I must have been forced to set my fist against that idiot's at least fifty times that night.

The girls Tubby had spoken of were his recently divorced wife, Liz, and her niece. At least I think they were divorced, because over the next four nights that we were stranded in Oakland he only slept in the house the first. No one ever told us for sure and we never asked. The five of us jumped into his car and left for the ill-fated concert. The niece was eighteen and joining the marines. She was absolutely giddy with the prospect and I got the sense that all of life's mysteries had been answered for her the day she signed her recruitment papers. While she rambled on, like a school girl in love, about the endless strong points of a military commitment, Tubby would intermittently interject, shoving his big, square head toward the back seat as he drove, boasting about how great the weather is in Oakland. "Every day Costa, every day is just like this. Every day is beautiful in Oakland." His eyebrows would raise and his little eyes would bloom in surprise every time he said it, as if he still couldn't believe how fortunate he was to live in Oakland. "Every day Costa."

The concert was as unimpressive as expected, nothing more than a bunch of late teen, early twenties girls dragging their boyfriends to cuddle up next to and listen to mushy, pop rock blaring at them from stadium speakers. Mercifully it ended at eleven and as we walked back to the car I had high hopes for the night to end so I could wake up early, start driving north on Highway 1 and leave this ridiculous character, who seemed like he belonged on Seinfeld, behind us once and for all. No such luck. The niece had promised her boyfriend that she wouldn't drink, and now after two red bull and vodkas she was tipsy and afraid that her cover would be blown. We stopped at a diner so she could eat something to sop up the alcohol and sober up a little. Tubby was in rare form, drunk and gorging himself on ice cream Sundaes, including the two extra Sundaes the waitress brought to our table by accident. He polished off Liz and Costa's left over milkshakes. All the while a glazed, retarded schoolboy look of inebriation washed over his square face. Regardless it was an impressive feat of eating conquest.

When we got home Liz and her niece drove away. I now think to keep up appearances for Tubby because we were only slated to stay in Oakland for one night. Tubby immediately stumbled upstairs to pass out. Costa was on the porch smoking a jack and I ran past him to grab my cell phone from the car. An old, dented 1980s style red Jeep with two thugged out dudes rolled by. I nodded to one of them and he shot me a gold-toothed grin. When I got back to the porch we realized that I had locked us out of the house. We commenced to furiously bang on the door, desperately trying to rouse Tubby out of whatever booze induced slumber he'd fallen into. Not a sign. "Shit Costa," I said. "We may as well grab the tent and set up camp right here on the damn porch." As it turns out that may have been the best thing for us. After another round of pounding and screaming at the door Tubby thumped down the stairs and swung the door open in his underwear. Tomorrow we set for Highway 1 and the wonders of the great northwest.

I woke up while the house was still silent, meditated for a solid twenty minutes, then got up and started gathering my things. I'd only taken two small bags out of the car, one with my pills for the week and the other with my journal. I hadn't planned to write that night, but the dream in Tahoe had instilled an almost unconscious paranoia that I might lose it, so I had grabbed it on the way into Tubby's place without even thinking about it. I opened the front door and focused in on a stunning sight: an empty parking spot right where my beloved Honda had been not seven hours ago. I ran across the street and read all the signs, at this point praying the car had been towed, but the signs informed me that no infraction existed to produce such a convenient reason for the empty parking spot on the side of the road. A nauseous, punch drunk hollow spread in my gut as a strange mixture of disbelief and panic rose up inside me. I sprinted back to the house and woke Costa up. "The fucking car is stolen, malaka," I screamed at him as I shook him awake.

"What? What the hell are you talking about?" Costa asked as he rubbed his eyes and focused in on me lurching over him like a crazy person.

"It's fucking stolen, man. The car is gone." The car and everything I had taken with me for a summer on the road had vanished. I still couldn't believe it. It sounded so bizarre when I heard myself say it.

Costa hopped out of bed and ran out to the street to check the signs, coming back with the same dumbfounded expression I'm sure was plastered on my face. Tubby sauntered down the stairs, his slumber no doubt disturbed by our frantic, early morning rumblings. "Is there any chance it was towed?" I asked Tubby, still working my way through denial.

"No way man, it was stolen." There was no hesitation in his response and I wondered if he had known that our car was in danger that night. The question flickered, but was snuffed out before I could think about it. There was too much going on. As I heard him call the police and report an auto theft I began taking a mental inventory of everything that was in that car and now gone: all my clothes except for one change and what I was wearing, all the camping equipment, my camera, guitar, most of my medicine for the summer, 600 bucks that I'd foolishly never deposited after a poker night in DC, my passport, even my fucking shoes for God's sake. It was a pretty extensive list.

Costa and I sat on the porch staring at an empty parking spot just the size of a four-door sedan. We were shell-shocked. The traffic buzzed from the highway and the crickets chirped in the trees, but all of it only served to frame that empty parking spot. What do you do when you lose your car on a road trip? "Well, the monks really fucked me this time," I tried to joke, "last summer they took my two thousand bucks, year before that my shorts, now they take my whole fucking car." The previous summer, coincidentally in Lake Tahoe, I had dropped a two thousand-dollar roll of cash on a day hike. That neat little bankroll had represented the money I'd won in shady home games across DC in the months leading up to the summer and was willing to put on the line that night in the casinos. Of course that never happened, and some hiker probably shit his pants when he came across two grand on a hike right behind me. On some level the whole thing was so ridiculous that it was hilarious, but the sting was too recent and the humor came out forced. I mean, who loses their car on a road trip? Tubby bounced out, with that square grin that seemed really out of place now and slapped Costa on the back,

"How 'bout this weather. Isn't it amazing? Every day it's like this, everyday is beautiful in Oakland, just like this." *Is this guy really going off about the weather right now?* I wondered, leering at him from the corner of my eye. I couldn't even look at him when he asked what we were going to do with our day, "Well whatever it is make sure you enjoy the weather, isn't it great. Everyday man, I swear it." I said nothing, afraid that if I answered I would quickly degenerate down a slippery slope of curses and meanness.

"Yeah Tubby," Costa muttered sullenly.

The police showed up soon enough, officer Benny Ayola, who as it turns out had loads of practice dealing with car theft. "Do a lot of cars get stolen around here?" I asked him. He laughed sadly, lifting a clipboard filled with two pages of stolen car reports from the last two nights alone. I filed my report and was told that if my car didn't show up in the next four or five days that I'd probably never see her again. Hearing that almost felt like hearing of a death in the family. I know it sounds silly, a car is just a car, but that car had been everywhere with me. I'd roamed the span of the country five times with her already and started to look upon her the way people see their pets. Yes you can replace your dog when it dies with a new puppy, but it's not the same. I'd grown so comfortable in her.

"The ninety-four to ninety-six Hondas are very popular with car thieves," the officer explained. "They're dependable cars and really quite easy to steal. All you got to do is jam a screw driver in and they'll start right up." When the cop drove away I sat back down on the porch steps with Costa. Both of us stared blankly ahead, bewildered as to what our next move should be, trying desperately to fight off the empty feeling that all was lost. I got to thinking about all the car thefts the cop had told me occurred in the neighborhood and how Tubby had lived there for fifteen years and I began to ask myself, with a fair amount of indignation, if he should have warned us. The question stewed inside me. At first I wanted to be better than blaming someone else for my problem, for in reality I should have taken the precaution of unloading the car myself. But it was too easy to blame him. Perhaps he could have offered us his driveway so the car would have been out of sight. I never even wanted to come here, shit Costa didn't either. Now revisionist frustration ran rampant through me. Costa had been half strong-armed, half guilt-tripped into coming to this God forsaken place and now my sweet, magical chariot of the road was lost. I started a Tubby bashing sentence, and then tried to catch myself, but it had gained too much momentum and I blurted it all out to Costa in quiet, agitated Greek curses that cascaded from my mouth in a poetic fury. No one can curse someone like a slighted Greek. He nodded meekly and solemnly agreed with every point and I saw that he was in a tough social place, somewhere Costa hates to ever find himself. A middle-aged woman walked past and asked if we had a car stolen. We nodded.

"Well I run the neighborhood watch and any car around here without a club on it gets stolen, I sent an email to all the residents about it." I shot Costa a look of disgust as she walked away.

I asked Tubby to take us to some pawnshops to see if any of my stuff had ended up there and he begrudgingly consented. I must admit the fact that he didn't want to do it added a vindictive appeal to the whole affair. The greatest populations of pawnshops are always in the worst parts of town, and so we drove to the slums of Oakland. Tubby waited nervously in his car, eyeing possible escape routes as Costa and I went into several pawn shops, swinging for the long shot of actually retrieving anything from this disaster. Clusters of sinister looking men with an air of aggression and general not giving a fuck-ness latent in their every action, look, and posture cluttered the door steps, smoking, drinking or plotting their next heist. We were quickly disregarded at everyone except the very last where the owner earnestly wished us the best. The exercise proved to be fruitless, except for the sole victory of irritating Tubby, which counted for something at that point. We gave up and were dropped off at the car rental place. Luckily I had full coverage insurance, so I was offered a free rental by the agency. Nothing came easy that day, but after a two and a half hour bureaucratic ordeal we finally got into a new rental and drove toward the Bay Bridge.

The car rental agency gave us a new, white Ford Focus. Getting into it felt like some kind of betrayal. Even though the car was more than a decade newer, and probably nicer, I couldn't find a comfortable position behind the wheel. It was foreign and wrong and really served to nail home the point that the Honda, my trusty companion on all my previous trips across the continent, was gone. The past is stubbornly unchangeable, and as we drove toward San Francisco Costa and I decided to continue with the trip, deciding that a realistic best-case scenario would be to leave on Tuesday, either in the rental or the Honda if it turned up. It was Saturday and we had to wait for the work week to start so I could go about the business of getting a new passport, a bank card and a whole new set of meds. If the Honda was retrieved we would go on as planned, dropping Costa off in Seattle and leaving me to drive to Austin from there. If not we'd ride to Oregon in the rental, loop back down to Oakland and leave in nine days by plane. I would fly to Austin and travel Mexico with Lobo, while Costa would go back to work in DC. Once in San Francisco we drove aimlessly, stumbling upon a park that was perched way up on a hill with a grand, sweeping view of the white city and the foggy bay. It would have been a great moment, a time to breathe in the shrouded city the way a bird does, but now it served as a distraction. When we grew tired of the wind we walked down and drove to Haight, walking around the hip degenerates of our time.

The prospect of seeing Tubby was less than enticing so we stayed out later in order to avoid him. The drive over the bridge, back into Oakland, was quiet and somber. The great spark of the moment had been extinguished in both of us and we were running on fumes, too obstinate to give up, but too drained to get properly excited. The street lights whirled by as we entered Oakland, land of car theft. I was caught by surprise each time they flashed upon this strange white car that I was driving, with an odd white hood and odd, unfamiliar panels inside. Liz was awake when we arrived and told us that Tubby wanted to take us to brunch the next day, to which Costa gave a tired, non-committal answer. Tubby was asleep on the two-seater, curled up awkwardly like a child. The three-seater was left for me and Costa's stuff lay on the guest bed upstairs. When Liz went to bed and didn't wake Tubby to join her I started to realize that their relationship was not what they were selling it to be. I would have felt sorry for him had I not been so preoccupied by my own troubles, a man nearing fifty, squished into a two-seater for the night in a house he'd lived in for fifteen years. But my thoughts were on too narrow a scope to think about him then. He wasn't there in the morning; God knows where he went to crash for the night. "Do you want to go to brunch?" Costa asked.

"At this point we have to take all the free meals we can get," I said and it was settled. That night *The Big Lebowski* aired on HBO. I'd seen it many times, but watched it again. The car theft scene meant a whole lot more to me now, and I got an ironic chuckle at "The Dude's" exasperation upon discovering that his clunker had been stolen.

The next morning brunch was scheduled for 11:30. Costa and I got up several hours earlier and did some pushups, which was the first time since I'd stumbled out to that empty parking spot that I'd seized the moment and made it mine. During the previous day I had turned into a car theft victim zombie, sleep walking aimlessly through bewilderment and self-pity. Such feeling is nonsense and I knew it, but it would come and go until I left Oakland for good. The brunch was nice, a 25-dollar treat of crab cakes over eggs Benedict, at possibly the only decent place in Oakland, the docks. "Man," Tubby started, chuckling to himself as he went on, "you're seeing so much of Oakland pretty soon you're not gonna want to leave." Horribly forced laughter spewed out of his mouth uproariously as he punched me and Costa several times to emphasize his point. He continued like a merciless butcher, "I mean is this weather nice or what?" At one time screaming, "what car. What car, huh guys, can you believe how nice it is out here today?" Each comment was callously delivered and completely out of context. It's almost like the man had bowling balls flying out of his mouth, all of which landed squarely on my groin. By this time I had wholly accepted that Tubby was a douche bag of the highest variety and would look off into the distance as if I'd heard nothing, allowing Costa to think of some diplomatic way of answering him.

That night our aimless ventures through San Francisco led us to the wharf. I battled with the sour taste the loss of the Honda left in me, trying hard to make the best of what's around and rise above the loss of mere materials. I couldn't tell what Costa was thinking. He seemed deflated, worried that it would ruin the trip, forever staining it as the time Nick lost the car he loved rather than the month we had the time of our lives out west. He was a trooper, paying for everything while I waited for a new bankcard. My passport needed to be replaced, which I hadn't thought much of yet. Cassandra called from Austin and informed me that if I wanted to travel with her and Lobo I needed a passport because the policy had changed and your driver's license was no longer enough to get into Mexico this year. She gave me the number for the passport agency, and so the agenda for the next day was set.

When I called the number the next morning I couldn't even speak to a human because of "record-breaking passport applications." The automated voice told me I could only be seen by appointment, but I couldn't speak to anyone to make one. There was no choice other than to drive down to the passport agency in San Francisco and see if I could talk to someone there. If I couldn't find a way to get a new passport issued my trip to Mexico would go the way of the Honda and vanish in the streets of Oakland. We got there right when the building opened and I was able to sneak by the entrance door unnoticed, the very entrance where a guard stood checking appointments later in the day. Maybe the guard had yet to arrive, or maybe the guy simply went to the bathroom, either way it was a lucky break. Costa drove around the city, and unbeknownst to me went on a mini Vittas shopping spree, buying me some much-needed shoes, socks, underwear and t-shirts.

The waiting room was rank with the stench of sweat and anxiety, not to mention impatience and frustration. Once I was in and could explain my situation the people there took pity on my appointment-less soul and directed me toward the correct line to stand in. I started talking to this lady I had held the elevator doors open for on the way up. She was middle aged, with short sandy hair, a big mouth and a flat nose. Her face had more wrinkles than her eyes would lead one to believe should be there, which were warm, still sharp with a twinkle of youthful playfulness. She had a big broad smile, and flashed it sweetly, like a mother, when I told her of my car troubles, telling me that her son had an old Honda and it had been stolen three times, retrieving it twice, "so you never know what might happen," she said with a wink, "you may get it back after all." Before I could let the ember of hope flicker inside me a younger kid, probably in his twenties jumped into our conversation.

"Where'd you get it stolen at?" he asked.

"Oakland," I answered.

"Oh, you ain't never gettin' that thing back. I had my car stolen out there, never saw it again." All in all the whole passport application process was far less painful than I had anticipated and after a quick four hours I was told to return the next day and pick up my brand new passport. Costa actually had to run in and pay the fee, 217 bucks, but paying for my stuff was apparently his new cross to bear, next up my lunch. On the way out the lady with the broad smile finished her book and gave it to me, which was fortunate because all the books I'd planned to read this summer were in the car, along with everything else.

We walked out the front door and saw a line stretching around the block to get into the passport agency, with a guard carefully confirming appointments on a clipboard. How I got in so easy I'll never know. After lunch we strolled around the city until we came upon a park by the bay. As Costa and I lay on the grass it occurred to me that we were losing days of adventure to idle, lazy hours in the Bay area. These aimless, meandering treks through the city were exhausting because they were destined to be fruitless. There was no purpose other than to kill time; wait for the passport, wait for the bank card to arrive, always waiting for some miracle involving the return of the Honda, but when you're acting as time's executioner you only drag the whole affair out. It was time to do a little dragging right there, so I plopped my head on my pack and began reading as Costa dozed off, curling up with his pack in the shade. Then like a gunshot this guy started screaming directly behind us. His face was flooded with a peculiar rancor and raw, youthful, undirected anger bellowed from his voice. He had crept up on us, pacing several feet behind us, screaming in song, "I love marijuana, I love marijuana, if you love marijuana, let's smoke some marijuana, now, hey. I love marijuana." He was young, with scraggly brown hair, dirty, white sweat pants and an equally dirty white shirt. He stopped right behind us for a verse, blaring his bizarre message for all the world to hear, then marched on, spontaneously breaking back into his song as he went along. His words were harmless enough, it was their delivery that was threatening. I tried to stay calm and see what he would do next, remembering times when I had done similar things when I was his age, not really directing my anger at any one individual, but rather displaying it in public, as if to tell myself that the days when I would cower beneath the public eye were gone. I sensed the same thing in him.

"What the fuck was that about?" Costa asked. "Let's get out of here," he cried as he sat upright, surveying the land for the next attack.

"Relax," I told him as I tried to explain where I thought the kid was coming from. But I had to admit that, aside from the lady at the passport agency, it seemed the whole bay area was against us, like we were the focus of some mass conspiracy and the entire region could converge and swallow us whole at any moment. Later that night we wandered over to the baseball stadium and scalped a set of nose bleeds to the game. Neither one of us is much of a baseball fan, it was just something to do, another way to drag time over the coals of existence and avoid the house on Vernon Street for one more night. The wind had been sucked out of our sails, and momentum proved to be a difficult thing to build standing still in the Bay area. I knew when my bank card arrived and I could get a new set of meds and we finally left this God forsaken hole of robbery and stagnation the events of the weekend would recede like a distant story endured by weary travelers of another era.

"You got mail Nick," Costa excitedly hollered the next morning. It was the long awaited bank card and we immediately drove out to REI and bought some six hundred dollars worth of camping equipment, all of which I would keep, but half of which Costa paid for. His sad, woebegone eyes, doleful to almost comic proportions by the rug swept from under their feet look since the car was stolen were starting to sharpen with the notion that perhaps this trip could revive itself. We cut through the city with a fair amount of acquired precision to the passport office where I picked up my new passport a mere 27 hours after beginning the process. That's got to be some kind of bureaucratic record. My passport photo was perfect. "Look at this shit Costa, tell me this doesn't say it all," I proclaimed, showing him the picture.

"Hell yes," Costa agreed in between laughs as we studied and dissected this unsuspecting piece of art that captured our moment in time perfectly. It told the story of the lost car, and the douche bag who we'd stayed with and the fucking Goo Goo Dolls, the whole story in one tiny two by three inch scrap of paper. In the picture I had a beat, stepped in shit glaze over my half shut eyes, a thick stubble growing on my tanned face, my hair was a mess, and a slight curl of the left half of my lips betrayed the self deprecating acceptance of the exhausting humor that the situation undeniably possessed. It was "The Dude" to a tee, straight from *The Big Lebowski*. What else could I do but abide.

Darwin's Grin
September 28, 2009

"A tree that is unbending is easily broken."
—Lao Tzu

*E*very time the pain comes back I get deflated. It's been a long road. I've been at this for over a decade and I'm tired of persevering. I'm tired of exercising patience. There were years in the middle where I was so close to being healthy that the only things reminding me that I wasn't were the medicine I took every day and the fact that I didn't drink or smoke like everybody else. And in a way those years of relative health almost make it harder when some part of my body starts breaking down and hurting again. It's like climbing until I'm several feet from the peak of a mountain, but then perpetually losing a foothold and tumbling back down. I don't want to give the impression that I'm not grateful for those years when I was near the top and everything was easy again, because I am. But each time I slip down the mountain I wipe out another route up the damn thing and a gnawing frustration builds because every time I got so close I put my guard down, and it felt so wonderful to put my guard down. The carefree novelty of enjoying a jog, or a weekly game of basketball, or slouching on the couch without worrying about all the possible repercussions of such reckless abandon never wore off. And having to re-raise my guard is just as big a burden as moving through the day in pain.

Usually the first few days I deny it. I try to ignore that my legs have begun to ache again, or that my head and neck are so stiff that keeping still hurts, yet moving around hurts even more. I choose to disregard the fact that I can feel the blood rushing through my head because each pulse feels like a tap from a hammer. Or I try to push through, ignoring the fact that my back is so tight that every breath comes with a stabbing twinge below my shoulder blades, and that even though I'm moving at a cautious, deliberate pace each exhale is deep and pronounced, as if my lungs are trying their hardest to expel the hurt that throbs with each step I take. But the thing that I really try to block out is the knowledge that this pain, whatever pain it may be, is here to stay for a long time. It's something I can feel in my body, as if the pain has somehow carved a niche deep inside the muscle tissue of the afflicted body part and only time can slowly erode its grip. So for a while I naively wait it out, hoping it will be gone in a few days, but the truth is I know with an aggravating, intuitive persistence that I'll be dealing with this particular episode for much longer.

Part of the initial denial ritual is this sludge that comes up all around me, around my thoughts, around my body. I mope along, trudging through it, walking down the street as if I'm wading through mud. My mind also feels like it's operating within a swamp. Thoughts labor within my head in slow motion, subdued by the numbness I bring upon myself to stave off facing the situation. At these times I try to detach myself from everything, from my hopes, from my dreams, from the present moment, but most of all I try to detach myself from the pain. This numbness has a short shelf life—somewhere around several days—and is shattered the moment aggravation propels me to wish. Once I start wishing there's no going back, the spell of malaise is broken. *I wish my head didn't hurt so much. I wish this God forsaken tension would leave my back. I wish my legs didn't throb as if I'd just run a marathon every morning when I wake up. I wish I was healthy.* The wishing phase is even shorter lived, usually just an instance of weakness, and is so obviously fruitless that it tastes sour in my head and I spit it out immediately. If I learned anything in the years before my diagnosis it's that wishing only leads to more wishing. I know that such thinking is the first step down a road of aimless suffering. Nothing good ever came to me from wishing, so I banish all wishful thinking. This part, at least, has become easy.

It's funny too, because in some ways when the pain is more severe it's easier to deal with on a mental level. When it's really bad there's no room to brood and ponder how much easier life could be, there's only coping with the present moment. Once I've pulled myself out of the malaise and have some clarity to my thought and, for example, have become ready to face the fact that the muscles of my head and neck are so tight that a cannonball might as well be anchored to my forehead, all I can do is breathe to get to the next step, then breathe again to get to the step after that. The pain grabs my attention and brings it to my breath and I start to meditate on the air rushing in through my nostrils, on my diaphragm swelling out then drawing back, on the rising and retreating tide of my lower abdomen and everything else dissolves except for the present moment. The greater the pain the stronger gravity my breath possesses. Gradually a strange thing happens: I come to peace with the pain. I accept it as part of the here and now and try not to put a value on it because I'm just living from moment to moment to moment to moment. I begin to notice that even though I hurt, there are parts of life that are not a challenge. There are still things all around me that come warm and easy. Trees still sway in the breeze, their leaves shimmering like ballerinas in the sun. The blues still makes my world swing, just like it did yesterday when my head felt fine. A tender, stoic pocket still glows inside of me, just like it always does when I focus on it.

When I really fall back deep into the rhythm of my breath I still feel the pain. It still hurts, and I still have to dig inside myself and find the strength to continue on with my day at work or at school or at a friend's house, but I don't fight it or hate it and it doesn't eat at me emotionally. Wasting precious energy glaring at the pain under a negative spotlight only serves to feed it and deplete me. Observing the body I inhabit and its sensations, along with the world I inhabit and its stimulants, I feel and don't feel, I'm connected and unplugged, I expect nothing and quietly persevere, gliding from moment to moment. It's not easy and I don't always find this rhythm, but when I do, my burden is lightened by its inherent composure. By yielding to the pain I overcome it. By accepting it, I can move past it. By acknowledging the physical limitations the hurt places on me, I see them as temporary. My breath is my guide and I humbly follow it to peace in the mental calamity that chronic pain can turn into.

But there's still another balancing act to accomplish: seeing the stiff neck, the aching back or piercing headache as temporary, I try to keep one foot grounded in the realm of peace and acceptance and the other firmly planted in the arena of faith and determination. It is attune to simultaneously focusing your vision on the road you stand on and the road ahead. It sounds like a contradiction, but it's more of a compromise, a flexibility to be able to incorporate two belief systems without washing one out with the other. And in this game flexibility is key. I say all the things I've been saying for years: *I have faith in God. I am loved by God. I have faith in my body. I am going to be healthy. Nothing will stop me from being healthy. All paths lead to my health.* But it is important to note that these words, these mantras, these affirmations are not framed within the context that life is unbearable or even unsatisfactory until I attain health. They are spoken behind the steady tempo of my breath, with the notion that possibilities are infinite so why not reach for what I feel suits me best? By no means is my happiness attached to the day that I rid myself of this disease. My happiness is not rooted firmly to anything.

When facing adversity I have discovered that your happiness must evolve. Your happiness must be open to morphing itself into an idea that can fit into the constantly changing conditions of your life. Carl Sagan tells us that life requires a delicate balance between mutations in DNA's nucleic acid and staying the course. Too high a rate in mutations and eons of well crafted, evolutionary inheritance is lost. Too low a rate will leave the organism overly susceptible to changes in its environment. It's the same concept with your outlook on life, which is really, at the most basic level, your perception of what makes you happy. If you tamper with your view of what constitutes joy and fulfillment too liberally, you run the risk of erasing the foundations of who you are at your core, ultimately losing a lifetime of accumulated beliefs. Some would argue that might not be such a bad thing, but not everyone is ready for such a drastic release of their ego. If, on the other hand, you remain rigidly attached to one specific set of circumstances that must occur in order to be happy, you only succeed in increasing the chances that your happiness will be suffocated by the limits that you have placed upon it. Think of your happiness as an animal—to give it the greatest chance of survival, you must give it freedom to adapt and bend into the different shapes that changing circumstances demand. Thinking that you can only be happy if you are healthy or if you start a family or land a successful job only places your happiness one step away from extinction.

In many ways your happiness must be like water. The ancient Taoist philosopher Lao Tzu has a fascination with water. One gets the sense that he spent countless hours sitting on the banks of streams and rivers, contemplating the contradicting properties of the water rushing by. In chapter 78 of the *Tao Te Ching* he observes that, "Under heaven nothing is more soft and yielding than water. / Yet for attacking the solid and strong, nothing is better; /It has no equal. /The weak can overcome the strong. /The supple can overcome the stiff." I think he sees the ability to adapt and change as water's greatest attribute. It always flows toward the path of least resistance and immediately takes the shape of whatever contains it, deferring to the structure of a bowl, a river, or an ocean. You can place a boulder in front of a stream and the water will simply flow around it instead of stubbornly clinging to its previous path. Some may see this compliant characteristic as a weakness, but over the course of time, if enough rain falls that stream will wear the boulder down to a pebble to be swept away by the current that hardly noticed nor cared the boulder was ever there. Lao Tzu sees great value in the ability to yield. To me yielding is the basis of evolving. You must surrender to move freely. Surrender doesn't mean giving up, but rather relinquishing excess baggage that won't let you survive the changing times. In this case the excess baggage would be any rigid concept of what you need to be happy because as Lao

Tzu says, "Green plants are tender and filled with sap. / At their death they are withered and dry. / Therefore the stiff and unbending is the disciple of death. / The gentle and yielding is the disciple of life."

Today my neck hurts. My head hurts. My face hurts. I'm so damn tired I can barely move and even the dimmest light comes at me like I'm staring at the sun. I'm trying real hard to focus on my breath, to focus on all the good things but it's hard when the bones above my eye sockets feel like a truck is resting on them. If it were possible for a truck to be resting on the back of my head at the same time I wouldn't be surprised. Noise blasts from the TV as if I was sitting front row at a metal concert until I turn it down so low that I can't hear it at all. Standing up to wash the dishes becomes its own accomplishment. Once the momentum starts rolling I pull it off without a hitch. And the funniest thing is that I feel this way because I got bored yesterday and took a 20-minute swim at Barton Springs. I guess it's better than having no reason at all. After the dishes are drying by the stove, there's nothing left to do but breathe. I take one deep breath after another and a shy grin forms on my lips. It's not exuberant. It doesn't shine or light up a room, but it's there.

Happiness is not dependent on something as fickle as the absence of pain.

And We're Off
June 14–15, 2007

The school year was wearing thin as the end of May 2007 rolled by and we approached the middle of June. A great tension built inside me and all the idle chit chat that comes along with being a teacher began to crawl deep under my skin and I wanted to scream to all of them, the teachers and parents, to shut up, then run and take a bounding leap into the Honda and embark once again. The Golden coast of the west, the evergreen peaks of the great northwest and the deep mysteries of Mexico called out to me in pictures and visions and a magnetic pull in my soul. Each day dragged on slower than the last. Not very Buddha of me Jack would mockingly say. But then again, Jack can be an asshole.

Finally on the fourteenth of June Jack, Costa and I were heading west. The Honda was packed to the roof with all our shit. The plan was simple enough: We would haul ass to Zion National Park in Utah where Cristina, Jack's girlfriend, would meet us. She would be driving from L.A. She had recently decided to move into Jack's mother's attic in DC. Jack would jump into her car and they would start their trip back east together while Costa and I would continue north, through California, Oregon, and Washington, ending in Vancouver. Costa would then fly back to DC from Vancouver because he had the incredible misfortune of not being a teacher or an online poker player, (Jack's chosen profession), and could only scrape away three weeks of vacation. From Vancouver I would drive all the way to Austin and meet up with Lobo and together with his wife and son we would all drive into the depths of Mexico for a solid month. The plan was simple enough, and actually destined to be carried out, though in a really roundabout and slightly bizarre way.

Costa slept in the back seat, surrounded by bags and my guitar basically resting on his head in the rear windshield. I drove and Jack sat shotgun. We commented on how this was the third summer in a row that we were heading west for a trip. I felt a great deal of pride in this and hoped the streak would never end.

Like Costa, I met Jack on the high school basketball team and continued a friendship from there. Jack Flynn is an athlete, in both mind and body. He's almost obsessively competitive. He is also pale as a ghost and heavily freckled, relics from his Irish roots, and has a set of shoulders so broad that they almost fold in on his chest, as if his chest just can't hold the weight of his frame and caves in on itself. And he has a unique way of fending off boredom too. Basically Jack produces a barrage of unending sarcasm. It's all slightly self-deprecating, but also filled with a healthy sense of reserved arrogance, leading to a string of judgments that relentlessly fly from his mouth. I buy into it and play the fool rather often, and we pass hours laughing at the ridiculous ramifications that my actions imply.

We drove into the night. I lay my arm down on the armrest and brushed up against his. The first time he moaned in disgust and lashed his arm away. The next time it happened he lit into me. "Why can't you move my arm away like a man, why do you have to brush your arm hairs all up against mine?" he demanded. "You know, we might as well just start sucking each other's dicks."

"Spare me, you want me to do it because you keep putting your damn arm where my arm is going to rest."

"I can't help it if my forearms are just so massive they take up all the space in this tiny car," he shot back, admiring his arms like the body builder he wished he were. "When I started going back to the gym I told you I'd be buff by August... well it looks like August came early this year." I made a gagging face at him. We sped through the night and went on in this way. And through a series of round about tangents, touching on many previous issues one held with the other, it was established that Jack and I would be carted next to each other in our times of dying.

"And there you will confess to me that you always agreed with every spiritual, hoo doo voodoo' comment I made, you always believed that monks up in the Himalayas can heat soup with their hands and walk through walls." Jack rolled his eyes for this particular point always irked him.

"The ones that took your shorts?"

"Yes the ones that took my shorts because I was too fond of them." I continued my rant, "and you'll say, 'Nick, I always agreed with you, I was just too hard headed to admit it.' And then I will turn from my deathbed to your deathbed and tell you that I understand, and that I forgive all the egregious assaults you threw at my character. Then our arm hairs will bristle against each other's and in an act of repentance you will admit your love and admiration for me. Then we'll both walk toward the light."

"Shut the fuck up," Jack screamed in between muffled laughter. The yelling roused Costa from his back seat slumber.

"What the hell are you two bickering about?" he asked still half asleep.

"All right trick hip," Jack fired, referring to Costa's bad hip, "first of all you're embarrassing yourself, no one can take you seriously right now sleeping beauty. Second of all if you were staying awake like a man and had to listen to the bullshit your fellow Greek immigrant has been spouting off you'd tell him to shut the fuck up too, trust me." On we went until somewhere in Ohio. We drove six hours that night, due to a late start, but the real driving would begin the next day.

We made Hayes, Kansas our destination and built all our efforts of locomotion on the simple foundation that after seventeen hours of readjusting ourselves in the same tired, cramped space we would get to collapse on beds and have the content dreams of heroic, driving champions. We arrived in Hayes, bleary eyed and stiff all over and saw that precious foundation crumble. Every motel in a town of motels was sold out, and the next town was full and the next. Jack and I had experienced a similar, bizarre lack of vacancies in Reno the year before. We had started in Denver and similarly placed all our faith in finding a room in Reno, but were unable to find lodging until we passed Sacramento, three hours down the line. It quickly became apparent that no town within 100 miles of Hayes had any vacancies and we lumbered on westward for 130 miles until we found a room in Colby. All in all we spent twenty-two straight hours in the car, slept for five, then drove for another twelve, reaching Zion National Park in Utah late the next evening.

Through chance and miscalculation we found ourselves on the eastern side of Zion, far from the RV populous the town of Springdale offered down below. We got there way after dark and were the only ones in the campground that I could see. We scrambled to set up a fire, then huddled around its glowing radius and ate canned beef stew that warmed the desert night chill away. I ventured off to the Honda and lay on the hood staring at the black sky that was littered with so many stars they seemed to be crashing off one another. It was a twinkling, glittering, snowstorm of diamonds in the coalmine sky. I folded my arms behind my head and lay on the hood like a hammock, breathing in the starlight and the campfire and the muttering voices of my friends, and all of it nourished some hibernating spirit that roused in me and burst with gratitude, saying, "we're here, we've made it."

Crate Full of Blues
January 1999

Reality finally set in around the end of 1998 when I admitted that I was sick. I had to leave my friends in Umass and move back home, into my parents' basement, in hopes of finding out what was the matter with my body. My last weeks in the log cabin house we all rented, deep in the woods of western Massachusetts, were some of the wildest I've had. I smoked as much weed as I could get my hands on, then smoked more. I took acid two, three times a week. Sobriety was a thing to be avoided at all costs. I shoveled these prescription horse pill ibuprofens I'd been given by the campus clinic, and threw in a handful of over the counter Advil whenever that wasn't enough, all in an attempt to dull the pain. I was taking the equivalent of about 25 Advil a day. I still hurt, but with the pills I could push the pain far away enough so that, sometimes, I could pretend that I didn't feel it.

After coming to grips with the fact that things weren't working, and that I had to go home, I wanted to enjoy one last indulgent run in Umass; the kind my friends still hadn't even thought about giving up yet. And so I did, to the best of my ability. Tripping with chronic neck and back pain can be a hard thing, but I was determined to push through for some childish reason, and usually the worst of the pain came the next day anyway.

When I left Umass I didn't pack a bag. I left everything there except a crate full of blues CDs, a quarter pound of dirt weed stuffed in my jacket pocket, and a ten strip of acid. The acid was for a friend who was waiting for me at the Greyhound station when I arrived. He was gone in a week. Everyone was gone. I found a job at a video store down the block and gutted out 40 hours a week as I went from one doctor to another on my days off. I bitterly concluded that loneliness is the stubborn feeling that you're stuck in a place you don't belong. I felt like I was stuck in a body I didn't belong in too. Where were Lobo, Dre, and, Kyle? Where were Matt, Johnny, and Mark? Five hundred miles to the north. And what madness were they basking in? I could only imagine as I walked the daily route from home to store, and back again, and winter turned to spring.

All my friends were away at college, or working bullshit jobs with general ease and disinterest. They were all juicing the mad recklessness of their youth whenever a spare moment arose, joyfully burning the candle at both ends. I was left to work the video store late shift and shuffle between one doctor, who didn't know what was wrong with my back and neck, to the next. I worked from five pm to one am. At times my back or neck would seize up and the job would be arduous, but I kept at it until my legs began to hurt in the summer of 2000—that's when everything fell apart. I'd usually smoke a joint on the walk home, arrive nice and high, and try to forget where I was. There was only one thing that really soothed me at those times: that crate full of CDs.

I'd been introduced to the blues two years earlier when someone had given me a Howlin' Wolf tape. I can mark my life in two separate sections, before and after Howlin' Wolf. I listened to that tape and was moved, felt a seismic shift within, as if a chunk of my soul had dropped down to this newly discovered depth of emotional intensity. I didn't want the tape to end. I anxiously dreaded the click the tape would make when the album was over. I immediately flipped it over when it did and heard it again, and again, and again. *This* was for me. This sound resonated inside my guts throughout the day. Long after I'd stopped listening, I was still listening. Quickly I jumped into the blues and amassed a little collection.

At home, in the wee hours of the night, after I'd left the fluorescent buzz of the video store, I went to my preachers. I sat in my room, put my headphones on and listened. John Lee Hooker, Muddy Waters, Lightin' Hopkins, Little Walter, Freddie King, Robert Johnson, Johnny Winter, and Howlin' Wolf became reverends of soul and grit to me. I listened to their every word and intonation. I listened to the way their instruments wailed and strutted simultaneously. I listened to a raw level of emotion that was clearly transmitted through crackling, old recordings. I felt a great connection to the music, as if this raw sound was, not only relating to my life, but digging deeper within my soul, mining so far into me that it was creating new emotions for me to experience. The music not only related to my experiences, but went past that, allowed me to feel levels of depth and intensity that the artists created for me to feel, depths I'd never touched before.

Every night after work I walked home, put on my headphones, and went to church. The inspiration my preachers, Son House, Mississippi John Hurt, Duane Allman and the rest, gave me was real, much more real than any fool standing on a pulpit, because the blues moved my insides. The music was simple, but rich with so much substance I'd often have the almost orgasmic feeling of too much emotion flowing through the too small hole my heart had to register it all—like a river running through a nozzle, exploding in a violent spray on the other side. My body was the other side, whatever was roaring through my soul reverberated through my whole body. The sensation wasn't a high, it was more of a low; it was deep.

I passed my nights in solitude with the music in this manner. The music became an entity that awaited me when I got home. And though I couldn't express myself to it, I couldn't vent to the music or engage the music the way I would a friend, the blues was something I could get lost in and evolve in too.

Miracle Blue and the Patron Saint of Recklessness
July 12, 2007

Lobo's wife Cassandra had taken Junior and their new Toyota Matrix over to San Antonio, leaving Lobo and I to cruise around Austin in his beloved "Miracle Blue," the legendary heap of beaten parts and bolts that still motors from point A to point B through some form of divine intervention or mistake. It's an 86' Volvo that he bought off a craigslist ad, showing up to his meeting with the owner with 1000 bucks stuffed in his pocket and 200 more crammed in his sock. When the owner scoffed at his 1000-dollar offer, 500 below the asking price, Lobo miraculously found another 200 in his boot and polished off the deal with a crooked grin and a firm handshake. It may be the best 1200 bucks anyone's ever spent. When he got a job building houses with our old landlord in Massachusetts he hauled that thing from Austin to Boston twice in one summer. The thing just keeps going. He's been driving it now for six years without a problem. The old Volvo makes ungodly sounds when it shifts gears, has lost its front grill, the lights work when they feel like it, but it still goes, the road's own little miracle. The car was in worse shape than when I saw it a year ago and got progressively worse every year I did see it. It rested on four mismatched tires, one of which was a donut Lobo had been driving on for a solid two months. This donut was beyond worn down, completely tread-less and so smooth you'd think it was made of porcelain. It threatened to burst at any moment.

"Volvo, engage," Lobo demanded as he turned the ignition. His wide nose snarled as his eyes, that somehow almost always held at least a tinge of drunkenness, bulged in a pleading grimace. The motor grumbled and moaned then stalled out with a shiver, sending a tremor through the entire frame of the car. I rolled down my window to let some air in. It was dreadfully hot, and even though I had no doubt she would eventually start up, I knew we could be waiting a while. "Ha, ehhh?" he laughed as if he were embarrassed, then tensed over the wheel like the car just might jump into light speed and screamed "Volvo, engage," while turning the key. His wiry shoulders trembled and his dark eyes squinted under the weight of some psychic effort he exerted. The motor sputtered and wailed and sadly stalled out. I've never seen the Volvo start before at least three warm up runs. The third time proved to be the charm and the old motor rhythmically grumbled as we made our way to the store. We approached a red light and were surrounded by a group of nicer, newer cars; by newer cars I mean cars that weren't cruising into their second decade on the road. "Quick, roll up your window so people think we have AC," Lobo blurted in a panic, frantically rolling up his window as we approached the light. We were out in the middle of a brutally hot Texas afternoon and I knew he was kidding; but I never know for sure. Perhaps he drove this old heap around by himself, sweltering with the windows closed, smiling out at his fellow commuters as sweat poured down his face.

"No," I objected.

"Oh, Okay. You're right," he relented with a half wink. "Now let's get some food for the ride, we've got a long trip tomorrow." We were slated to leave for Mexico the next morning. The only thing that kept us was the arrival of our friend Dan and his girlfriend.

Dan and Linda were arriving by bus from Boston that night at an incredibly inconvenient time, right in the middle of a blues show Lobo and I were both excited to see. Around seven we sat at the bar listening to the warm up acts hoping the headliner would take the stage late enough for us to catch most of his set. All week Lobo had been going out to shows with me with the understanding that he would "drink like a gentleman," which meant refraining from boozing all his money away and ending up black out drunk. Requesting such restraint is a hard thing to ask of him, but one that was necessary because he'd already gone on his standard pre-vacation pawnshop run and there was no more money coming in until August. If we were to go to Mexico he couldn't afford to squander what meager funds he had on a bar stool before we left. But enough was enough. Lobo was working on his fourth beer when he informed me in no uncertain terms that he would not be drinking like a gentleman on this evening.

"When I get drunk I like to steal shit," Lobo told me with an emphatic, boisterous chuckle as we raced north on I-35 to the bus station. His Aztec face popped in and out of the shadows as the Volvo labored by street lamps at a lumbering 75 mph. "I don't know why that is," he continued, reflecting with a smile, "but I just wanna take shit when I get drunk. Like this one time, I was hanging out with this guy and his father, real Austin big shots. The dad was boys with Stevie Ray Vaughn and the son dated one of the Bush twins. We got wasted and ended up back at the father's house and I went to take a piss in the backyard and the old man ended up getting' all pissed at me and we ended up gettin' into a fight right there. Nothing major, just a scuffle, you know, some pushing and shoving and rolling around. Somehow the kid gets into it and I swiped his phone as they were throwing me out. In the morning I'd forgotten that I stole it, and the phone was ringing in my pants when I called him. He's never wanted to hang out with me again," Lobo concluded laughing with sick, heartfelt, glee as we pulled into the bus station.

As we drove away from the station Lobo squinted his eyes, darting quick glances around, muttering to himself, "this doesn't look familiar. Are we sure we're still on thirty-five...yes, yes, yes, we're still on thirty-five, but this all looks unfamiliar." Dan asked him if he'd been going north to get to the bus station because we were still heading north now. A goofy, embarrassed look swept over his face and we u-turned south. He pushed the motor to 80 mph to make up for lost time. Lobo was mad with excitement over our friend's arrival and the show and the impending trip. He started frantically rattling off his own personal tour of interstate 35 as we sped through the night, toward Antone's and the blues. "Right there, that's where I worked for two months when I first moved down here. I got fired for doin' whip-its in the kitchen. Me and my buddy Damon killed every can of whipped cream they had in the place. They were holding some promotion where they were spraying these bare-chested, contesting chicks with whipped cream and every can they grabbed was dead, and just leaked milk on the chicks on stage. One after the other, they kept trying cans and all of them were dead and the chicks were just holding their tits up on stage and didn't know what to do." He started laughing, but interrupted his laughter to continue. The motor roared up to 85 mph as the dashboard trembled. "Oh, right there is where I go to work out." He spun around in his seat, whirling his meaty finger at what he wanted us to see, seemingly looking anywhere but straight ahead at the road, but the car kept right along. The mood in the car was joyous and relaxed. No one thought, hey this guy should be looking at the road instead of Dan in the back seat. "This is where Cassandra and I ate dinner once, it was okay, this is where I bought some pants, this is where I farted once two years ago, it smelled pretty bad." No detail was spared. The tour continued into Austin until we arrived at Antone's right after the first song. Dan and Linda had no idea the peril they were just in, I had lost sight of it.

The next day, rolling up to a drive-thru, the long used and abused donut finally gave out, basically tearing in two as we idled to the window. The damn tire split open as if someone had taken a knife to it as we drifted up to the teller. Lobo popped open the trunk, pulled out the original, full sized wheel which had been flat for a couple of months, hoisted it onto his shoulder and sauntered down the street to a tire shop that just happened to be across the parking lot. He ambled along with that old full sized flat resting on his shoulder, as if he had waited for the most reasonable time to change the damn thing. As if everything had gone according to some detailed plan of his. I waited under the shade of a tree and it occurred to me the danger we must have been in as we raced up and down I-35 on that threadbare, old donut, which was defying physics by merely staying intact. Had we driven another mile at that speed the tire would have surely ripped open on the highway and who knows where the car would have ended up. It didn't occur to me how dangerous this was but I seem to lose sight of such precautions when I spend time with Lobo. It's almost like he has the patron saint of recklessness watching over him, always one step ahead, preventing countless catastrophes from erupting on a daily basis. You start to feel that by being with him the saint will cover you too. The patron saint of recklessness has taken note of his life, fallen in love with the way he lives it, and vowed to always protect it.

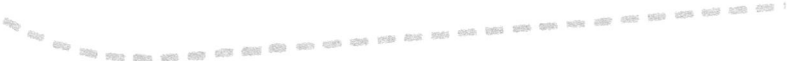

The Missing Makes It More
March 1999

Hours drag by in the video store. I've become friends with a group of Africans that I work the late shift with, Ebou, Mamour, and Joe. We call him Joe because he says his name is too hard for Americans to pronounce and he doesn't like to hear it butchered all night long. Ebou and Joe are tall and lanky, while Mamour is short. They make fun of his height incessantly as Mamour grits a forced smile that is filled with dreams of vengeance. Well, we're kind of friends. I don't see them outside of the store, but at least they make the time go by a little faster as we work. Most of the time they don't say anything about whether they notice if I'm in pain or not. Once Ebou said he wished he could help his friend who was suffering, and once Joe commented on the fact that I never bend over, wondering if it affected my lovemaking.

I'm lonelier now than I've ever been. My entire crew of brothers are up north in Massachusetts and I'm stuck in DC. Dealing with the bizarre, unexplained way my body is breaking down is hard enough, but doing it without any friends around is that much harder. I hadn't realized it before my health started failing me, but so much of my identity was tied to my friends and my athletic ability. I've lost both now, and kind of have to start all over. I've got a lot of time to think about things these days, so I'm coming up with all sorts of insights that do me no good.

I miss my friends. I miss having people to carve laughter into the day with. I miss being part of a group, a mob really. I miss basketball. I miss basketball dearly. The basketball court was a place where I could lose and reinvent myself. I had some talent. I could shoot a jump shot better than anyone. I could fall into a rhythm and stroke in one jump shot after another effortlessly. I could fall into a zone for a month, and scarcely miss a shot the whole time. I wasn't the quickest, or strongest, but I had a will to win, and an ability to get that jumper off when someone quicker and stronger was doing all they could to stop me from doing just that.

Most nights I smoke a joint on the walk home from the store and fantasize about playing again. My heart flutters and races as I picture myself draining a pull up three in traffic or a contested fade away from the elbow. That euphoric intensity, which is unique to basketball, surges in me as I watch myself whipping a crisp cross court pass, or stuffing a block on a breakaway, because even though I can't jump, I got long arms and good timing. But all the fluttering, racing, euphoric intensity is a diluted sham, and I drink it nightly only because I'm thirsty and have nothing else to drink.

The NBA season is rounding the corner and the playoffs are approaching. I tape the national games on Tuesday and Thursday night while I'm at work. When I get home I smoke another bowl or two and get real high, high enough so I can almost forget the last couple of years, high enough so that if my neck and back start hurting I'll be too confused to feel sad. It works sometimes. Often I'm so fucked up I forget to fast forward through the commercials.

I watch these games now with more intensity and passion than I ever did. I have an almost perverted interest in them, like a virgin watching porn. I take note of every detail of every play. I rewind plays to study the looks on the players' faces. I scrutinize their body language before a play transpires, gauging the strength of some hidden, nameless force that drives them to succeed or fail.

In the commercials that I forget to skip I start to agonize over the sport. I wonder how sweet it would be to play again, how wonderful it would be to feel that swelling pride that sets you floating when you hit a game winner on game point and everyone knew you were going to make it before the ball left your hand. I think I'd be as free as a bird if I could get that back—nothing could get me down. Now I'm just stuck here thinking about it, and the images fester upon themselves and go rotten in my head. A couple of years ago if a roadblock surfaced in my life, I'd go to some lonely court with street lights and shoot jumpers until I was lathered in sweat and my mind had been wiped clean. And even if the resolution to whatever problem I had didn't materialize, there was the solace of an empty mind. Now the roadblock is the inability to go shoot and the frustration builds into mounds.

I woke up to the symphony of roosters crowing and donkeys braying to the new day. The tent was already balls hot so I got up and tried to catch a little shut-eye on the hammock attached to the side porch. I attained mixed results until Lobo burst out of his room and any ideas of sleep were carried away by his booming voice bounding around the house. He was excited to be back in La Madrid, land of his family's roots, deep in the arid, mountainous wasteland of Mexico. We were down for a weekend, staying in his mother's house, which was packed with numerous relatives visiting from Texas, other towns in Mexico or just down the alley. I was the only one there not part of the De Los Reyes gene pool. "Hey V," Lobo thundered as he bounced around his mother's porch, speaking to me in between sets of calisthenics, "you wanna go check out the canyon behind those mountains?" he asked me, pointing over to the dark peaks that cut into the horizon to the west.

"Sure," I said, "let's eat first."

"There's no time, pretty soon the sun will start cooking," he said as he approached Belli, a gangly 14-year old cousin of his down from the closest city, Monclova, who was dutifully trying to stay asleep. Lobo looked a lot like Belli before the creeping onset of middle age added some beef to his frame and face. But he was still rather slender, and in great shape, and made an issue of walking around shirtless as often as possible so the world would know. "Ven hijo," Lobo roared and gave him a swift kick. Belli rubbed his eyes for a second, put on his boots and was ready to go. The three of us jumped into "Miracle Blue," the legendary heap of scrap metal on wheels, and off we went.

Lobo, Belli and I headed to the corner store, one of only a handful in the village of La Madrid, where we bought a loaf of bread, two avocados, and some cheese. We swung by Gordo's house to see if either of the two eldest boys wanted to come with us. Paul came out barefoot and shrugged his consent but Lobo sent him back in to get some shoes because we had a lot of hiking to do. "She drives like a dream, huh Vittas?" I looked down at my feet, which were surrounded by sand, to the point where I thought I was in a sand box. The glove compartment was completely ripped out and I could see the gizzards of some part of the electrical system. The car let forth a whimpering wail as he switched gears. "You know one summer I drove this bad boy from Austin to Bar's place in Massachusetts twice. I was so broke I slept in rest areas the whole way up, and I had no rear windshield because this dude smashed it in an act of revenge against me for pissing in his Jeep. It was a great time. I was by myself on one of those long drives and the radio's never worked in here so I started making up raps to pass the time," he laughed and pounded the dashboard. He displayed some of his freestyle skills. They were horrible.

We drove away from town, toward the big green mountains that ring the village. Soon the road deteriorated, as if we were driving on a dried up river bed with huge rocks and massive holes laying in it like an obstacle course. The road only got worse, and Lobo's eyes sharpened with focus as he swerved the car from side to side to avoid these treacherous boulders and pot holes that threatened to end the Volvo's miraculous run and leave us stranded in the middle of nowhere to roast in the sun. He skidded to a halt right before a ledge almost a foot high where the road dropped like a step. We all got out and pondered the next move. Lobo asked Paul if we'd have to walk from here, but that was out because it was another 40 minutes by car. The idea dawned on us simultaneously to create a ramp by placing smaller and smaller rocks against this natural step. The four of us jumped to it and we were barreling down the road in no time. From here on out I rode on the hood and the two boys on the trunk because we had to continuously hop off to remove boulders from the path. As we drove through the canyon I sat on the hood looking up at the huge green mountains. Their jagged peaks pierced the blue sky and beautiful dark green creases fingered down their steep slopes with the hot sun baking the metal hood and me as well. Every five minutes we'd hit a bad stretch, either littered with boulders Lobo couldn't maneuver around or a really steep incline that the Volvo couldn't conquer with our added weight and we'd jump off the car then scramble back as we bounced and rolled on down the road. His eyes grew maniacal with focus behind the wheel and I knew that he had decided that he was going to drive old "Miracle Blue" to the very end of the road unscathed. His driving was determined and masterful. His eyes, blazing in the here and now, found every turn, avoided every obstacle like they were lit up with neon flashing traffic lights. At times we'd hit an open stretch and he'd rev the engine up to 35, 40 mph and I'd have to hang on for dear life, as he still had to swerve around an occasional rock.

And here lies the beauty of traveling or just living with Lobo; you have to trust him to take you to the edge and not lead you off the cliff, and in turn you're forced to trust yourself not to get hurt because you have to dig inside and find the fearlessness he has to pull it off unscathed. This occurred to me as I was holding onto the windshield wipers with a clenched, white fist, bracing myself on the hood with my legs as we raced down the rocky, bumpy, swerve-riddled road. We sped down every straight way we came upon. It felt great on the hood of the car, almost like I was riding a motorcycle, maybe even better as the charging wind rushed over my whole body, as if I was flying through the canyon. The lunatic behind the wheel began to needlessly swerve into oncoming bushes, laughing uncontrollably over the roaring motor as Belli, Paul, and I were forced to plow through the branches. No doubt the patron saint of recklessness was laughing too.

We got to a point where there was a three foot step separating the road from the trail and Lobo proudly pulled the car up next to several trucks that had made the trip. "Trucka, trucka, trucka," he boasted the comparison, pointing at all the trucks and laughing with his younger cousins. We hiked down the trail, which grew narrower and more overgrown as we progressed, until we came upon a stream that was fed by an underground spring. I knelt down and splashed the water on my face. It was an offering of sorts as much as a moment of refreshment. I was grateful to be feasting on the bread of the moment. We followed the stream. Around was the thick brush of the arid mountains, rich with shrubs, cactus, and small trees. The stream led us to a waterfall plummeting from a small cliff. The water roared through the exposed roots of a tree that seemed unable to decide which level to settle upon and chose the middle ground, then pounded down onto smooth, yellow rocks and ran off into the stream. A group of loud kids were drinking by the falls so we followed Paul, who said he knew where the source of the spring was. We climbed up a fiercely steep hill, tromping through the thick underbrush until we reached an anti-climactic hole gurgling clear water down toward the falls. Lobo wasn't impressed, and insisted that there had to be another source, but Paul knew better, though he didn't offer much protest when his elder cousin started marching further up the mountain.

Paul was hard to read. I couldn't tell whether his stoic, calm eyes portrayed an incredible, timeless maturity or if he was just a shy, reserved ten year old. There was a composure about him that's rare to see in a child, like he'd seen it all before so nothing was really worth his excitement. In some ways he was in direct contrast to Lobo. He was our ten year old, grandfatherly guide. And he was tough too. He was the only one wearing shorts as we weaved our way up the mountain full of disdainful plants intent on sticking you with countless spikes or thorns. We reached a rundown barbed wire fence, rusty and evil looking. Lobo and Belli hopped over it pretty easily and as Paul was contemplating his mode of attack I reached back and lifted him over like the babe he really was. I couldn't tell whether he was grateful or insulted, probably a bit of both. The terrain became angry, almost reproachful as any remnants of a trail vanished and we pushed through the arid wilderness until Lobo was satisfied that no other pool lay up this side of the mountain. Paul gave no hints of self-righteous indignation, though he had been right. We sat on the toasted rocks that lay in the sparse spaces in between the cactuses and shrubs and ate the avocado and cheese sandwiches that Belli doled out. They were dreadfully plain, but delicious at the same time. We sat there as a warm breeze stole some of the power from the glaring sun, a grand beautiful mountain towered directly opposite of us, and the stream was little more than a tiny ribbon of silver way down at the bottom of the canyon. I pulled my hat low over my eyes to block the sun's glare and let my body rest while my soul bathed in the glowing feeling of peace that permeated everything on the mountaintop.

On the way down Paul muttered something to Lobo in Spanish. "Paul says to watch out for charging bulls," he nonchalantly translated. I didn't really know what to make of this comment. It could be some stupid joke or I could become an unsuspecting matador around the next bend. "If a bull charges at you run to the nearest tree and keep going around in circles until it loses interest," Lobo advised me over his shoulder. Either this joke was being beaten to a pulp or there was a very real possibility of coming across a wild bull out here. Apparently there were wild cattle roaming through the canyon and with wild cattle came wild bulls. The four of us casually made our way down the mountain until we came upon an open plateau and everyone immediately tensed up and quieted down. In front of us, directly next to the only path down the mountain stood a massive, hulking, white bull. I glanced at it for a second, then ducked my head and tried to calmly scurry along without exuding fear. As I followed them past the bull, which gave a snort as we passed, I searched the landscape for a tree to run around, but only saw one tiny little weed of a tree within running distance. When I looked at the bull, all I saw were those two longhorns shooting out of the side of its big head. I never looked at the bull again, but I could sense its mammoth presence behind us as we slowly and silently made our way past it.

"Did you see that thing?" Lobo asked me, wide eyed with excitement like a boy.

"Did I see that thing, what the fuck do you think, how could I not see that thing?" I told him. He spun around and went through the same exchange with the boys. Belli shared my sentiments, Paul was far more reserved, only admitting that yes, he had seen the giant, wild bull we walked five feet in front of. We made it to the edge of the cliff unnoticed, climbed down to be met by another bull not five minutes later as we walked by the stream. This one was farther away from us and scampered away when Lobo and Paul yelled and threw rocks at it.

The stream was shallow but moved fast and there were nice deep pools where we could submerge our bodies. These cool, refreshing natural tubs were heaven sent to our sun beaten bodies and all four of us stripped to our shorts and laid down on the smooth, water worn rocks which had perfect back rests built in. After a half hour or so we headed back to the waterfall and thankfully the loud kids had moved their party elsewhere.

The waterfall was beautiful. Crystal green, icy water crashed down upon three distinct levels of rocks after plummeting from the original cliff face with the tree and its exposed roots hanging seemingly in midair. Paul and Lobo disappeared, though I could still hear their laughter. I realized that they were actually inside the base of rocks that made up the lower level of the waterfall. It was hollow. I found a small crack that seemed as much like an entry point as anything I could see. Taking a breath, I dove and swam to the dark. When I emerged I found myself inside an underwater cave with its own miniature waterfall splashing down in the corner. The water in there was freezing, being untouched by the brutal, Mexican sun. I saw Paul's narrow eyes glow with an exuberance that fit his tender age for the first time in the dark, crisp cave. Belli soon popped in and the four of us walked around in awe of the treasure we had just discovered. The jewels of the road are infinite. Bright light tore through a couple of cracks creating a dim, nightlight effect that allowed me to see their faces. We stayed in there until the cold water had seeped into our bones and we began to shiver, and then popped out to be toasted by the sun. After venturing in once more hunger overtook us and we began to hike back to the car.

But, the adventure wasn't over yet, we still had to navigate through the riverbed road that led us there. The jolliest of all Volvos was waiting in the dust for us. Lobo sat in the driver's seat with a tired resignation, preparing his mind for the focused determination the drive out of the canyon demanded. The boys hopped onto the trunk and I slid onto the hood and we were off. Lobo drove with more confidence now, racing down the straight ways even faster as I held on with all the might I could squeeze out of my knuckles. The wind screamed into my face, the embankments were a green blur, the Volvo's ancient engine growled with enthusiasm, and all the while the stoic, green mountains stood peacefully in the distance watching our tiny slice of madness. I thought to myself that if he flips this car I have to jump off and propel myself far enough to escape the rolling, blue carcass of metal that would follow. I knew he wouldn't though, and focused all my energies on hanging on. Every now and then I'd check to make sure we hadn't lost one of the boys on those sudden turns to avoid a boulder or a hole. They were still there, holding onto the sides of the car and grinning with dark eyes that glimmered in the daylight.

All went well until we reached a steep drop that led into a steep incline, like a roller coaster. We hit a patch of grey sand and the Volvo skidded to a stop. The back tires spun around in frustration, kicking up sand and dust, but the car wouldn't budge. A truckload of locals approached us and when the men of the family realized we were stuck they sauntered over to give a hand. Four of them, Paul, Belli and I pushed the Volvo, though I faked it because my legs were already aching and I feared a collapse if I pushed them too hard, while Lobo revved the motor to no avail. One of the men ran back to the truck and returned with a shovel. Lobo grabbed it and attacked the soil around the rear tires with a frantic, fevered, madness, like the key to life lay hidden in that dirt and only he could dig it out. He flung one shovel full of dirt after another, sometimes spraying the locals with a shovel full without noticing. He was completely engrossed in his job. The sun glistened off his back, whose muscles were grinding and pulling in mad spasms to the merciless commands of a man possessed. "Why don't you have one of us rev the motor and you push on the back of the car?" I suggested to him when he laid the shovel down. I didn't say so, but I felt that we could use his fierce determination there. He agreed, and with several rocks back and forth old "Miracle Blue" spurted out of the canyon's trap to the applauding whistles of the family waiting behind us. Lobo was embarrassed by the delay that his car had caused and quickly thanked everyone, then jumped back into the driver's seat and raced up the hill waiting for me and the boys to catch up and hop on. Riding in the car seemed boring now and we held on even as the riverbed turned back into a road, holding on all the way back to the house.

Lobo's madness is infectious. Or rather his fearlessness is. Somehow you lose sight of consequences when you're around him and all that's left is the excitement and the adrenaline and the subtle notion that no matter how out of hand things get, everything's going to work out. He inspires you to be reckless for recklessness' sake. Ridiculous propositions like, "let's climb up the fire escape of this college administration building, find an unlocked window and break in at four o'clock in the morning while we're tripping on acid," not only seem plausible, but inevitable, as if you owed it to yourself to, for once, act without fear. That's what Lobo pulls out of you almost by the sheer gravity his appetite for intensity possesses. Yes, the crazy situations you find yourself in when with him never have a tangible reward, and any reasonable man would tell you the risk involved far outweighs the jubilant excitement of being completely absorbed in the moment, but that's what being reckless is. It's the lust for that excitement that attracts the patron saint of recklessness to someone like Lobo, because it's those people that give the saint a purpose.

The Vermonter Runs North and South
April 19–24, 2000

*T*he Vermonter runs from DC straight to Amherst, Massachusetts in nine hours flat. It's not that long of a trip and the train seats are a lot more comfortable than the bus, even if a ticket is more expensive. That being said, it had been a year and a half since I moved away from Umass, Amherst and this was the first trip I'd made back to see my friends. For all of 1999 and the start of 2000 my neck and back hurt too much to come back. I felt the pain would keep me from enjoying myself, or rather would hurt me more if I saw how I couldn't enjoy myself. I was friends with a real rowdy crew up there, and times were never calm or relaxed, usually bordering closer to the brink of disaster than anything else, so how could I keep up with them if my body was in constant pain?

Come April of 2000 I was confident that I could handle a visit and I secured five days off from the video store and a ticket on the Vermonter. My body had been feeling slightly better for the last month, (though in three months I would hit my absolute rock bottom), and I was beginning to come to grips with the limitations that the, at that point, nameless condition, placed on me. The trip went well, all in all. There were times when my neck hurt so bad that I wanted to go hide somewhere. There were times when the group got real crazy and I had to step back and watch from the sidelines, carefully monitoring my body's aches, rather than screaming and howling like an animal with the rest of them. These moments were hard, particularly because I had been a spark plug for such occurrences in the past and now I didn't know what to do. But, I didn't have any completely overwhelming episodes of pain—the kind of pain that turns me into a zombie— and for that I was grateful.

The five days were up. I woke up early, weaving through the discarded kegs in the bathroom as I brushed my teeth. I found Lobo passed out on a couch by the deck, the rank smell of tequila wafting all around him. Traces of vomit and wing sauce stained his hooded sweat shirt—the good life. I woke him up and he drove me to the train station. We threw pebbles into puddles as we waited for the train. Lobo was too hung over to talk, I just didn't feel like it. "You got any weed left?" he muttered.

"I got this roach left from last night, but no lighter," I told him. Lobo got up and stumbled to the other end of the brick shack of a station, sauntering up to this dingy, dank, hippie kid smoking a cigarette. He hustled back with a little more urgency, waving the lighter in triumph, and I pulled out the tin that held my one-hitter and the roach. The dingy hippie followed Lobo and asked us if we had a bowl. "Right here," I told him as I opened the tin and handed the bowl to Lobo, who eagerly sucked down the roach in one greedy inhale before he was asked to share any. Lobo's eyes nearly popped out of his head as the hippie pulled out a big jar of bright green buds from his backpack. The kid had good weed, the whole platform stunk like a field of pot plants the second he opened the jar. He packed the bowl almost unconsciously, and then asked if I'd ever smoked opium before. "Out of this bowl or ever?" I said. My question to his question seemed to pose as an answer as the kid sprinkled a thick layer of opium over the weed, lit the bowl and passed it to me. I took a blast and let Lobo finish the rest.

The train pulled up and I got in, high as a kite. The last taste of the way I wanted to live floated out of my buzzing head, trailing out of the closing doors. I sat in my seat and the train lurched forward as the whistle blew. Tears built up on the corners of my eyes. The Vermonter runs from Umass straight to DC. I knew why I didn't come up there that often.

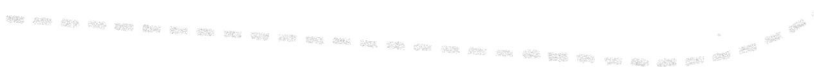

Baptism By Smith
June 28, 2007

We were well into our second day away from the Bay area, but the relief I had expected to instantaneously feel after we put Oakland firmly in our freshly rented, rear view mirror was only partially present. Losing the Honda had a hangover effect, and Costa and I were both a little skittish with our exuberance. It seemed that we couldn't completely let our collective guard down and enjoy the breeze of the journey for fear of the next slap in the face that may lay right around the corner.

As we turned inland, Highway 1 changed dramatically from a ribbon of asphalt tracing cliff lines on the shore, to a thick tunnel of trees and branches, with cracks of sunlight shooting down to the ground. Running up and down mountains we entered the "avenue of the giants," and were introduced to the Redwoods. These are the monks of the earth, anchored in the same plot for a thousand or more years, slowly reaching for the heavens with saintly patience. Stillness spilled from these giants and engulfed their forest, as if the whole thing was in a deep, meditative trance. Green life thrived in every direction within this jungle overgrowth. A cave of leaves hid the sky, and the ground was buried beneath a mossy carpet. Vines drooped down in zigzag patterns, and giant, dead logs resembled flowerpots as vegetation toppled over itself in heaps. A week ago a scene like this would have put me in heaven. Now I took it in with a modest appetite. I hated to admit it, but I was still reeling from the standing eight count Oakland had hit me with. I'd accepted the car theft, abided by it and even laughed at it, but somehow two days away from Oakland and I still couldn't quite shake it. I wanted to be carefree, completely electrified by my surroundings, but was buzzing at a reserved hum at best. A persistent hesitation dampened my excitement, and I felt as if I was going through the motions of what genuine zeal should feel like.

Just as we left the Redwoods we saw a stout, balding man with the remnants of a grey, bushy fro, a thick beard, and small, round-rimmed glasses, hitch hiking off 101. "Should we pick him up," Costa asked behind the wheel, "it'll be exciting."

"Sure," I said. We needed a jolt. When we pulled over the stout man ran over to the back seat and introduced himself as Ron in a high pitched, raspy, granola voice that reminded me of Jerry Garcia. The pungent smell of sweat and body odor wafted in with him and Costa immediately rolled down the windows. He was an interesting little guy, rambling on excitedly about the beauties of his land like a mad tour guide determined to get every point across in the limited time available.

"The Smith River is a world renowned river, it's one of, if not the cleanest, rivers in the world. You have to swim there, man. Well, really you've already blown it because late May is the peak swimming hole season and it's already late June, but it'll still be nice..." In this frantic manner he covered countless swimming holes and campsites we should visit, all of which I forgot except for Patrick's point campground. Costa and I snuck in a couple of questions when Ron would gasp for air.

"So, do you hitchhike often?" Costa asked him.

"Oh yeah, man, I've never owned a car," Ron boasted, "never needed one. I've always been able to get a ride somewhere, and if I can't get a ride back immediately I'll just shack up where ever I'm at and try the next day, but that rarely happens." It sounded as if Ron rarely had any problems working either, but I never got a chance to ask that question.

"Have you ever had any problems hitch hiking?" I asked him.

"Only twice in fifty plus years of thumbing it," Ron answered with a chuckle. "Once I got picked up by a drunk and was certain he'd crash and kill us both, but we made it all right."

"And the other," I prodded.

"The other, man, was in Hawaii. These two Samoans picked me up and after a while I realized that they weren't driving me to where we'd agreed, and even worse I knew they meant to do me harm, man. Have you ever heard of the powerful, puffer fish?" Ron asked, but he didn't wait for a response. His voice changed as he went on, falling deeper and deeper into a near growl that was laced with an unnerving intensity. "The powerful puffer fish can blow itself up to ten times its size when it senses danger," he snapped. "It can scare away predators by making itself look bigger than it actually is." I looked into the rear view mirror and saw Ron's face change from a harmless hippy to an almost bear like animal, with a mouth that snarled and menacing, bulging eyes. *Take it down a notch, Ron,* I thought to myself. "Well, when I realized what those Samoans were up to I blew myself up, blew myself up so those Samoans didn't think I was worth the trouble, and then I leapt out of the car, backpack and all, and they kept goin', man, because they didn't think I was worth the trouble after that, after I had blowed myself up so big."

And so Ron became powerful, puffer fish Ron to us from then on. The puffer fish gave us a little scare, but quickly deflated to his friendly, chipper self. We dropped him off at an exit on the side of 101 and continued to Patrick's point, arriving at the precious moments just before dusk. Costa and I huddled around a campfire and ate pork and beans. I could still taste Oakland in my food. That goddamned Ford Focus was an outrage, looking all new and white and void of any soul and character—the opposite of the Honda. *Those fuckers got my car, man.* I couldn't help but let that thought slip into my mind every once in a while, even if it was with a chuckle.

When I woke up the next morning I had a moment of clarity where I realized that a road trip is analogous to a life lived. Life is boring without a little adversity, and the car theft was our piece of adversity. Instantly my enthusiasm stopped being a precious thing I had to coddle and look after. We continued north on 101 and I told Costa that we should look at our travels like an adventure rather than a vacation. He dug what I was saying, rolling it around in his head for a second before proclaiming, "it's an adventure." It started to rain and we cut across to highway 199, through foggy northern California and into Crescent City, where we stopped for a quick grocery run.

Back onto 199, through the rain which varied from splattering sheets to a thick mist, and into the Smith recreation area, home of Powerful Puffer Fish Ron's beloved, pristine, Smith River. We turned off at Myrtle Beach, usually a popular destination, now deserted in the rain, and all the more beautiful for it. "You wanna go for a rainy swim?" I asked Costa.

"Adventure baby," he hollered as we parked the car on a turn about a mile from the highway. We changed into our trunks and scampered down the muddy, wooded trail that led to the river. We stood at the foot of the beach as the cold rain pattered down all around us. This was our first taste of the Smith River and it was wonderful. The water was perfectly still and fast moving at the same time. The color was a clear, fluorescent green, with patches of aqua, Caribbean blue mixed in. And when I say it was clear I mean perfectly clear, clear enough to see the individual crevices of the rocks 20 feet below, but with this beautiful, almost artistic green tint that the surrounding forests gave the river. It was clearer than air because its waters had no haze to sift through like the air above. An old bridge arched 100 feet over the water, which trailed off into green mountains. The mountains themselves disappeared into the low hanging clouds. We tucked our clothes under some bushes and walked to the small beach as the rain came down on our shoulders.

After some hesitation on the edge we dove in. The water felt as clean as it looked clear, and seemed to rush through me instead of over me. Diving into water that pure, that clear and simply perfect is an electric joy, a joy that slaps you in the face and sings, "see here, look at the beauty and wonder of your existence." I dove deep underneath, pumping my legs and cutting my arms through a cold that surged through me like a charge, that rattled around my core and lit some fire within me as it froze the flesh on my frame simultaneously. When I popped up to the surface, I swear, the grins on Costa's and my face lit up the whole forest. The swift current of the river had swept the previous week, and all its meager troubles, off us. The weight had been lifted off our backs and hurled downstream. The moment had once again been placed in our laps. Powerful puffer fish Ron had been our unwitting pastor, leading us to the banks of our sojourning salvation. Reborn and revived we eagerly anticipated what lay across the next horizon. The past was over with, washed away so far now that it may as well have happened to someone else.

With easy grins we continued with what time we had left. Plans of making it to Vancouver had vanished with the Honda, but we managed a quick loop around northern California and even made it to Crater Lake, Oregon, before doubling back and returning the rental in Oakland. Costa flew back to DC, while Lobo waited for me at the airport in Austin, screaming for a run through his homeland of Mexico. I was clean when I got there too; I'd been baptized in the Smith, after all.

An Introduction
November 1999

I'd been gone from Umass for almost a year now, and been sick for almost two. No one could tell me what was wrong with my body. My life had turned into a steady procession of fruitless doctor's appointments. I had managed to hold a job at the video store since returning to DC ten months ago, and that gave my time some form structure to build around, which provided me with a level of sanity. In the year previous to landing the job I had been concerned that the pain wouldn't allow me to work, so holding onto a job for that long at least alleviated some of the anxiety surrounding my future. If my body did not deteriorate any further, at least I could supply some sort of means for myself as a cashier. I had become adept at working in pain, and could push onward when the pain got bad, but I hadn't yet figured out how to live with pain. When my neck or back would hurt, that strange bone deep hurt, I would instantly become frustrated, angry, and most of all despondent. I felt that the pain was robbing me of my identity. I would curse and moan, and wish it gone, and constantly fantasize of all the things I would do if my body didn't ache so badly, so often.

One of the doctors that had no answers suggested I see a pain management therapist. I took an instant disliking to the therapist, finding her smug and patronizing. She made me expand on my answers in mind numbing detail, as if either she or I were an idiot and had to have every sentence explicitly explained. On the first visit she hooked me up to a heart monitor and some kind of muscle/ nerve sensor, like the ones that accompany a lie detector test. She led me through some deep breathing exercises in an attempt to show me how breathing affected all my muscles. At the time I was thinking, *if deep breathing could get me back on the court I'd breathe deeply until I passed out, other than that this is bullshit.* On the next visit the therapist led me on a guided meditation where I was supposed to picture myself on a serene beach or mountaintop, and this was supposed to alleviate my pain. It didn't. That was my last visit.

Several days later I returned home from a walk. I'd smoked a joint earlier but was just about sober again. I went to my room, sat down and decided to meditate. I'm not sure why I had this urge, but I followed it. Aside from the guided meditation I'd never actively meditated before. I didn't picture myself at a beach or a mountaintop, those kind of flowery images seemed fake and far from my reality. Instead I started to focus on my chest and quickly fell into the rhythm of my breathing, almost like falling into a comforter. I can't tell you why I focused on my chest other than the notion that that was where I felt the most alive. A reverberation emanated from deep in my chest. It was a vacuum to all my attention. I could focus on nothing but that reverberation as it started to spread from my chest and engulf my torso, and my arms, and my legs. I had this amazing feeling of being elongated out of my body, as if the reverberation was carrying me upwards. I was in my body, but also slightly above the body that I felt seated in the chair. It was a high unlike any I'd tasted before. At some point my focus lapsed, almost like it was too good and I just couldn't bear it anymore. I opened my eyes.

I tried to meditate the next day, and the day after, but didn't attain a similar sensation. Over the course of the next 12 years I gave up on the practice and returned to it several times. Each time I returned to meditation it was with the belief that something profound lay within the practice, and that belief stemmed from my introduction.

Enter Lobo
April 1997

"Hey, my name is Azel, but people call me Lobo," he told me. *I'm a person*, I thought to myself, *I'll call him Lobo*. Apparently some prick in the third grade had been unable to pronounce Azel and proclaimed, "I'm gonna call you Lobo," and the name had stuck. Lobo was a short, dark Mexican with a broad nose that he got from his Dominican Grandmother. He had uncommonly wide shoulders on his wiry frame. They hunched over his back in bunches of muscles and tapered off into an almost comically thin waist and scrawny legs. Umass had offered him a track scholarship that he promptly refused in order to party properly. Loans or scholarships made no difference to him, so long as he wasn't paying for it now.

I first met Lobo at the University of Massachusetts early into our freshmen year. He was seventeen and one half roadrunner, one half Tasmanian devil. Like a whirlwind of flesh and curses he would spin into a room, tear the place up and move on. In those days Lobo was a highly sensitive instrument that was being over loaded with stimulation. Insults flew out of his mouth at every turn. He paced and jittered and had a way of circling around people as he talked to them. His eyes feverishly darted around a room and his body immediately followed, moving at the speed of sight. He sweated profusely wherever he went. He sweated so much that he took three or four showers every day. Someone asked him why he showered so much and he gave some ridiculous answer like, "they're not charging me for showers, so I'm going to get my money's worth," but that wasn't it. The atmosphere had him running on overdrive. One day I went by this girl Maybelle's room, a cute little Ecuadorian chic whom half the guys in the dorm had made a play for, and I saw Lobo sleeping alone in her bed, heaving great, voracious sighs as a pool of sweat formed around him on her sheets. I remember thinking, *Jesus; this guy is restless even in his sleep.*

To tell the truth he was hard to be around during that first semester. He couldn't contain himself and the tidal wave of his persona felt almost oppressive. He seemed like a vindictive standup comic hepped up on speed, and was little more than a blur of hyperactive, nervous convulsions, cracking jokes and hurling insults at anything in his field of vision. "What, what's the matter with you, you're like a tree, you just stand there and say nothing. Shut up already, you're talking too much," he'd berate someone standing quietly in the group of a room he just burst in on, "and you, what are you gonna smoke that whole joint to yourself or do you think Good Ol' Bo can take a puff," he'd complain, grabbing the joint from the perplexed hand of someone who never even had a chance to say 'come in' or 'who is it' when their door knocked. He'd then walk out of the room and it wasn't until everyone started yelling that he'd realize, "wow, you mean that joint was still in my hand," with a guiltless smile.

It wasn't until he slowed down, or I sped up, or probably some combination of the two, that I started to realize how liberating his influence could be. And the liberation comes with the understanding that you have to allow his moods to move in swirling, unpredictable patterns. You can't count on him to be reasonable or compassionate, but you can't predict that he won't be either. I've seen him bend over backwards, exerting ridiculous amounts of energy to help a stranger. Then again I've seen him condemn his mother and brother several times. He once banished them to the shed behind his house when they teamed up against him during a family squabble, then taunted them from his porch. "I'm the big bad wolf," he howled, "I'll huff and puff and blow that shack down." Later, to really nail the point home he threatened to unplug the extension cord that lit up the little shed. If life was a movie he could play the villain just as easily as the hero.

What it comes down to is that you can't count on him for anything but to be a living, breathing manifestation of the here and now. Lobo has mastered the art form of extracting every ounce of substance from the moment and so an intensity defines every moment around him. It was my job to take that intensity and make what I wanted with it.

The night I first took acid was when I started to realize all this. It was the end of the semester and a near riot broke out on campus. I'd been up the hill in Van Meter Hall, drinking Whiskey with this guy we called Burma. Back then we'd developed a practice of scraping together enough money to buy a handle of cheap liquor and downing one shot after the other until the bottle was empty. Chasers were a luxury item. On this night Burma had given me about fourteen shots, which for my meager tolerance meant I was trashed. I stumbled down the hill in a stupor and basically rolled into a throng of at least 1,000 belligerent kids amassed on the steps in front of Gorman Hall. One of the houses across the street had hosted a party that was wildly out of control. The cops came and the crowd just screamed at them in one unified roar, like an animal. I swayed and weaved through the lurching bodies until I felt someone jerk my shoulder backwards. I turned and saw Lobo's face leaning into mine, his dark eyes bulging out of his head in excitement. "Kyle and Matt took acid," he screamed over the roar, "I know where it is, let's go take some."

I didn't respond, I didn't have time to or need to. The instant those words hit the air we ripped through the crowd and into Gorman Hall and flew up the stairs. I don't remember touching a single step, I was just soaring through the stairwells right behind him. One after the other, four floors disappeared in a flash. Kyle was Lobo's roommate and Matt was mine. We burst through Kyle and Lobo's door and Lobo started rifling through his roommate's belongings. Everything was moving faster than I could process. There was no time to think, there was barely time to react. I caught glimpses of Lobo madly cutting at strips of paper and shoving little pieces of paper in my mouth, and then cramming more into his mouth. His hands moving so fast as a fizz started to bubble in my head. Just glimpses. Just fragments of time that I caught as it all blew by. I have no idea how many tabs we took to this day; I just know that we took it all. The crazy thing is the moment he said, "let's go take some," we both started sprinting like a live grenade had landed at our feet. There was no debate, there was no discussion, it almost seemed like there was no choice.

When we came back down the cops were macing people on the front steps. Within minutes the riotous crowd had dispersed. Empty bottles and cups littered the yard, which now felt like a ghost town. We were both still drunk and staggered through the empty campus as the acid slowly overpowered the booze. Within an hour all remnants of the alcohol were gone and the acid stood front and center. In the nighttime everything glowed. The cracks stood out on the sidewalks like diagrams. A nervous, jittery twitch circulated through my body and an effervescent buzz drowned out all the noise of the silent campus. We smiled and giggled and walked like there were springs in our calves.

Down through the center of campus we strolled, up to the towering library Umass chose to set in the middle of their campus. I've always thought that Freud would have really appreciated the University's efforts to build the world's tallest library. We took a sharp left past the phallic monument and came across Old South College. It's an old, red building, probably one of the first ever built at the University. It looks very English-colonial, almost like a long row of three-story townhouses with a large five-story tower book ending one side. Every muscle in my body felt like a wound up coil, as if I was just bundles of tension reverberating off each other. The red bricks of the building started to glide into momentary shapes and faces, then fade back into their standard rows. I looked up and noticed that the stars are outlets that charge the night, give it an electricity that crackles beneath the surface of everything. "You wanna break into that building?" Lobo asked me. He said it so casually that it only seemed natural that we should. Shit, why shouldn't we.

"Sure," I said.

Never once did the notion that this wasn't a good idea pop into my head. Never once did any of the numerous possible repercussions enter my mind. Could we get caught, arrested, expelled? Never even entertained the thought. Were there motion detecting alarms waiting to alert the police inside? At that point it didn't even occur to me that they existed. Could I fall attempting to scale the roof and break my neck? The world might as well have been made of foam for all I cared. Nothing else existed except the prospect of entering that building. Lobo went up to the fire escape on the side of the five-story tower and started climbing upwards. Every move was fluid and decisive as he almost swung from one beam to the next. I followed behind him as he pushed up on windows to see if they were unlocked. The fire escape ended at a locked window and Lobo stretched out onto the roof of the three-story section, then scaled up the roof in a scampering, shadowy motion to a tiny window on the side of the tower at the peak of the roof. He pressed his palms up on it and it slid right open. I climbed up on the roof and crawled over the rough shingles, up to the open window where Lobo had disappeared into the darkness of the building.

The building seemed alive and to be peering in at us walking through its innards. We crept through the silent, dark halls and all I could hear was the thundering thumping of my heart beating against my chest cavity and an occasional board creaking with a piercing whine. How would I explain myself if we were caught? What could I possibly say? The idea never entered my mind. My eyes were bulging out of my head and everything in my peripheral vision swirled and glowed and crackled like silent fireworks. Every now and then Lobo would peer back at me with an ecstatic, beatific look of pure wonderment chiseled into his face. His eyes were crazy too. The outside world had ceased to be, and only the universe of the building existed and it was ours alone. Security guards to chase us had never evolved out of the protoplasmic goop that gave birth to life eons ago. Neither had cops to arrest us, or janitors to report us for that matter. There were no consequences in a world that consisted of nothing more than the two of us and the building. Still, we didn't dare make a sound, not because we were scared, but because it would have been sacrilegious to break the silence. We walked through a maze of disjointed offices and lounges until we came upon a mural painted on the full face of a wall. It leapt out at me and we were paralyzed before it. I can't tell you what it was a painting of because I never saw the painting, just the stunning, marvelous colors moving in such vivid, three dimensional patterns, literally leaping off the wall at me. I felt that we had been following a trail to this very mural all night and only just now realized it. Hallucinations took control of my mind and we slowly sat down and stared. This would have been the funniest position to get caught in, two wild men staring at a wall like it was a TV. I saw faces, animals, people, great, intricate scenes of life unfolding, and as in a dream I have no idea where they came from.

When it was time to stand up and leave we did. I couldn't tell you how long we spent there, only that the exact appropriate amount of time had passed. We walked down through a stairwell and toward an exit. Then a sound. A pipe banging? A security guard? The police? None of these concepts registered, only danger. I was filled with panic that rushed through my blood like a set of rapids, and we flew down the stairwell to the first floor, bursting through the door, then sprinting away from Old South College. For the second time that night I had the feeling of moving so fast that I was floating over the ground. I was faster than I'd ever been. My arms and legs pumped furiously and I cut through the night like an arrow. My breathing was calm, efficient, almost machine like. We were half way across campus by the time we stopped and crumpled into an uncontrollable fit of laughter that convulsed through me in waves of euphoria until my jaw burned and tears streamed down my cheeks and spit frothed around my mouth and the only thing that kept me from flying away was the ground. From that moment on I was pretty close with Lobo.

The Waiting Room
October 1999

I hate waiting rooms. I hate them with a passion. All the frustration of the last couple of years bubbles over when I'm left to sit in a stale room, littered with a collection of the most superficial magazines of our time fanned out on coffee tables like slices of thinly cut shit. It's 30 minutes past the appointment time. None of the staff say a word to me. No one shoots me an apologetic look. It's like they don't even notice me, or at the very least they don't notice the fact that I've been waiting for half an hour and counting. The receptionist won't look at me. The nurses who take an occasional patient to a second, private waiting room in the back won't look at me, and each passing second stews and simmers until my face is flush with disgust. What other business would manage its customers like this and stay afloat? None that I can think of. But these doctors have a monopoly on my health, they're the only game in town and they've got me in a vice because I need them. If there were a reputable witch doctor down the street that would treat me with a little respect, believe me, I'd be there.

It's mid to late 1999. I've been seeing one doctor after another, on and off, for almost two years. I left Umass about a year ago, and the contrast of my wild and rowdy existence at college compared to this waiting room, formaldehyde moment is enough to make me laugh—or cry. I've seen doctors all over the DC area, even flew out to the Mayo clinic once. All the meetings are pretty much the same. They go something like this. Doctor walks into the secondary waiting room that I've been placed in, at this point almost an hour late, absentmindedly glancing at a chart that I have to assume is about me. No mention of his/her gross lack of punctuality, not even an off-handed thanks for waiting. "So, ah, Nicholas, what seems to be the problem?" They ask.

"Well, almost two years ago I was doing some pushups and I felt a pop in the side of my head and my vision went white. Since then my neck has been stiff and really sore. Then, about a year ago my back started hurting, like a constant spasm that hasn't stopped either."

"Hmm. Is there any relevant medical history in your past?"

"I had Lyme disease when I was eleven years old."

"Yes, I see that," scanning my chart, "what were your symptoms then?"

"I had muscle pain, fatigue, stiff neck, double vision, and Bell's palsy."

"Bell's palsy? Half your face was paralyzed?"

"Yeah, but it went away after a few weeks."

"And I see you were treated at Children's Hospital in eighty-nine."

"Yeah, ten days of antibiotics."

"Mmm, that is a little short. Standard is two or three months treatment these days. No symptoms from eighty-nine to ninety-eight?" I shake my head. "Well, you've already had two Lyme tests in the last two years," the doctor concludes, "both of them negative." This is when the doctors abandon any connection to Lyme disease. At this point the best of them will run their hands over my shoulders and feel all the muscles bunched up in sharp, little knots. They'll find the hardest knots, the ones that feel like a packet of pebbles has been surgically inserted in the tissue and push on these pressure points that radiate painfully from the weight of their manicured fingers. When I flinch they give me a diagnosis of fibromyalgia, which is little more than a collection of unexplained symptoms grouped together with no real solution outside of pain management. Not only does this diagnosis take me off the one path that could actually help, but it's tantamount to doctors officially recognizing my pain and admitting they have no idea what its cause is. But hey, at least they're trying.

The worst of them start to ask irrelevant, patronizing questions like, "How were you doing in college? Did you really like it? Is there any possibility that you're just happier in DC, with your parents?" The worst of them will completely dismiss my symptoms, "You say your back is in spasm, but look how easily you can put your shoes on. I know a lot of people with real back pain that can't do that." The worst of them will fill their precious charts with the most unrelated information imaginable, like my disheveled appearance, or the fact that I have a handful of tattoos.

Lyme disease is incredibly complicated. Lyme disease is actually the bacterium Borrelia burgdorferi and was discovered in the early 1980s after a rash of unexplained illnesses in Lyme, Connecticut. The deer tick is the only vector, or carrier, of Borrelia burgdorferi, and the only way humans can catch the disease is from an infected tick's bite. This has all been common knowledge in the medical field for quite some time.

None of these doctors believe in chronic Lyme disease because they have no comprehension that Lyme disease has three distinct stages, not just one. In

90% of people the immune system or a round of antibiotics will catch up with Borrelia burgdorferi and eradicate it within the first two stages. For the remaining ten percent the disease becomes chronic, lasting years or even decades, with alternating cycles of remission and relapse. Old symptoms can persist and new ones can appear. These symptoms include, but are not limited to, muscle aches, fatigue, arthritis, memory loss, inflammation of cranial nerves, (resulting in the facial paralysis of Bell's palsy), mood disorders, heart arrhythmia, numb or weakened limbs, double vision, light sensitivity, and the list goes on.

The doctors I've been seeing for the better part of two years wouldn't think that I could still have Lyme disease because they don't know that Borrelia burgdorferi is a highly adaptable microbe that can shift its shape and alter its surface proteins to elude both the immune system and antibiotics for years upon years. The sick part is that most of this ignorance about Lyme disease exists because insurance companies are applying pressure on doctors not to treat the disease. These health insurance companies bring doctors who actively treat chronic Lyme disease in front of the medical board and make them fight to keep their license, ultimately scaring all but the bravest doctors from seeing Lyme patients, and perpetuating the ignorance and fear over the disease that leaves thousands of people to struggle with Chronic Lyme for years without the medicine that could help. But I don't know any of this useful information now either, and so I keep waiting.

A Mural of La Madrid
July 20, 2007

Almost every day around dusk I would grab the bike and roll around La Madrid, the tiny Mexican village of Lobo's ancestors. As the sun drops and loses its strength it throws gold on everything: the trees, their leaves, the farm animals, the meager buildings, the people. The air begins to grab traces of midnight cool and everyone, it seems, is out to enjoy the moment. Bike rides through La Madrid are the soulful, aimless, meandering rides of youth. Many times I see fellow riders gliding through the streets just like me. Some are children, faces beaming, racing, laughing, yelping like the overjoyed pups that they are. Some are old men quietly peddling along, beatific, tranquil smiles winking out to the world. Some are eager, teenage boys speeding down the alleys to play Romeo to their Juliet.

And then there's me, tall and gangly, I cruise around watching the movie reel of life in the village unfold before me. Two old Mexican cowboys converse around a horse. They're neatly dressed in jeans and button down, short-sleeved shirts. Their ten-gallon hats are pulled so low over their brows that all I can see is the shadow of their eyes behind the glare from the west. Deep wrinkles etch the passage of time on their brown faces as they smile at each other and into the mountains behind them. They nod to me as I pass. An old man, hunched over on his front steps, grins mischievously as he plays with his toddler grandson. He shoots a whistle my way as I roll by. Flocks of innocent teenage girls scamper by, dark eyed and mysterious. Mothers lean out of windows, screaming their children's names, and the called ones dejectedly veer away from their crew of barefoot rapscallions. A couple bickers in the darkness of their kitchen and a plate crashes against the floor. Scurrying feet patter across a field to the rhythm of a soccer game. One boy has a kick like a cannon and struts around the field like a rooster while the girls swoon. I can almost hear the silent, bashful blushes of his unofficial cheerleaders as he shoots a look their way after a goal. Men laughing, women gabbing, babies crying, children shrieking like visceral angels; all through the streets of La Madrid at dusk, a truly holy time.

And the dogs, the fucking dogs are everywhere. "You know why there are no stray cats in La Madrid?" Lobo asked me. "Because the dogs ate them all." At almost every corner a pack of stray dogs lie practically on top of each other, bold and unashamed, as if they own the block. Like gangs, they guard their turf and can be found on almost the same spots every night. Some gangs are harmless, moping fleabags. Others leap up and give chase. Snarling and barking ferociously they bite at my heels and relent only when they've forced me to cross some inner bridge of anger and desperation where I hop off my bike, convinced that this is the time I will have to fight these damn dogs. When they see that I'm ready to fight, when they see that they've dragged me down to their level, they smugly trot back to their posts. I started filling my pockets with rocks to whiz at any dog that needs a good pelting. These are the dusks of La Madrid.

But La Madrid is more than just fleabags and soulful sunsets. To me it is the birthplace of Lobo, despite the fact that he was born hundreds of miles to the south in the polluted metropolis of Mexico City. This tiny village, tucked discretely in a ring of mountains, is the perfect place for a kid to take his spirit out for a spin and see what it can really do. A boy can run wild here. He can tromp through dried up riverbed canyons that flood in a flash, and harbor wild bulls resting menacingly in the shade. He can race horses through dusty valleys, and kiss his cousins behind the cover of chicken shacks. The grand space can give an already reckless boy the notion that if he runs fast and mad enough only the mountains will keep him from soaring off into the pale blue open. La Madrid is a blended painting of the majestic and the mad. One of his aunts recently ran over her husband after an argument, and still feels entitled to call other people crazy. There are pieces of Lobo everywhere here.

I'm sitting on the porch of his mother's house when a pack of barefoot children slowly make their way down the gravel road. They kick up a plume of dust in their wake. Lobo, his wife Cassandra, his son Junior and I just got back from the wrestling matches in Monclova, the nearest city about an hour up Mexican highway 57. A pair of horses graze in the back yard. Lobo borrowed them from his cousin yesterday and has yet to return them. He's tromping around the yard between the two wells with a fierce squint in his eyes, running his fingers through his black hair in agitated sweeps. He's trying to get water to feed into the house, but it's no use, the pump simply won't cooperate. He takes note of the approaching kids. "Look, here come Gordo's kids, probably hungry and looking for a meal. Their father is a fucking retard. I mean I love him, he's hilarious, but he's got no consciousness. He fucks his wife and knocks her up, but after that he's all set. I've never seen him hug any of his kids. Shit, I've never even seen him interact with them or even look at them for Christ's sake. He'll talk to everyone's kids but his own." Gordo is Lobo's older cousin. He has a spherical potbelly and seven kids with a wife who's been pregnant for the better part of the last decade and has given up. The kids basically raise themselves. "Cha-Cha laid into their mother, 'why the fuck don't you take care of your kids. Why is everyone else taking care of them,' and all that. Which is true. Those kids will show up and won't leave 'til you throw them out the door. They follow the scent of food like a pack of dogs. Anyways, Cha-Cha said that and then their mother beat her down, shut her up real quick," he continues with a grin. He always loves a good fight.

Here they come now, at least the youngest six. The eldest has out grown such wanderings through the village. Their feet are like callused little boots. Kevin and Kenneth are seven and nine respectively. They are a pair of loud, obnoxious boys who love to mess with people. They see it as a sport to pass the time and Lobo breaks from his mission with the water pump to run after them as they walk up the short driveway. They laugh in taunting, giddy bursts as they scramble away and curse at him when he's given up the chase. Paul is our quiet stoic tour guide from the adventure down in wild bull canyon the year before. He's the constant observer, and smiles shyly as his younger brothers act like assholes. Mariana is thirteen and possesses a virginal sweetness that has an almost saintly aura. She's basically been a mother since the age of five. Jorge is the odd ball. He is darker than his siblings, and his face doesn't match theirs. The rumors are that he's not Gordo's son. People say the mother had an affair with the mailman around the time of his conception. It's not talked about openly, and the younger ones haven't heard this, but somehow they've caught on. Jorge is an outcast in his own family. The other kids shun him. Alana is the youngest, a three year old girl with a grown up scowl and a raspy, smoker's voice, the way you'd think a barroom angel would sound after a long night. She is the toughest of the lot and will scream, scratch and claw with any of the rest. These kids came to symbolize La Madrid to me, and since they represented La Madrid, they also served as a breathing mural to Lobo's writhing, lustful soul—at least the part of it that was bred down here.

Lobo berates them, asking them what they want, but they just deflect the questions and scatter about the yard. They're here for food and probably some break from the endless stream of fights that their parents entangle themselves in. Apparently Gordo and his lady really go at it sometimes. Alana strolls up to Junior and socks him in the face, then grabs the Dora the Explorer doll he dropped to hold onto his cheek. "God damn, that little broad is a real savage. This summer she was in the yard and she hiked her dress up, squatted down and took a shit, then got up and kept going where she was going, just like that. Squatted down and took a shit right in the yard, like a dog, not even a thought to wiping or nothing," Lobo told me laughing enviously. Kenneth and Kevin go to the basketball hoop in the back and Jorge shyly watches. They make no attempt to include him. Paul blends silently into the trees while Mariana smiles apologetically for their presence. Her tenderness is almost heartbreaking. It makes me silently pray that she finds someone, somewhere to nurture it.

Lobo goes back to his tinkering with the pump and I walk over to the hoop. Alana follows. "Callate, puta," I hear her mumble to the doll as she slaps it in the face. It's ridiculous to hear such filth fly casually from her mouth because she really is a cute, pudgy girl with big brown eyes and a playful little smirk on her dimpled face. That smirk can turn to a scowl as swiftly as the wind and it's not long before she overcomes her initial three year old shyness with me and is following me around, proclaiming, "tio, tio, juego comigo porque te pegas." I laugh because it's funny and endearing to hear a three year old threaten you with physical harm unless you play with her, but I can easily see her turning into the domineering aunt of the village, chasing kids around with a stick and shoving her nose in everyone's business.

I'm rolling a basketball back and forth with Alana. Kevin and Kenneth had been playing with it, but she commandeered it. Even though they could have easily wrestled it away from her, they felt it wasn't worth the battle that would surely ensue. Out of the corner of my eye I see Lobo sprinting toward the house, a mischievous grin formed on the corners of his lips. Soon he's running back to the far well with an extension cord trailing him and a small portable pump in his hand. He loops a garden hose around a tree, lowers it into the well, and has water running down like a shower. He calls me over, the mischievous grin now glowing broadly in triumph, having outsmarted the sinister fate that aimed to keep him sticky with the day's accumulation of sweat. "Hey Vittas," he hollers in excitement, "come check this out." The kids are following me to see what the commotion is all about. He lifts the iron lid off the well, which is nothing more than a concrete box filled with water under the ground, and lowers himself into the well. "Woo wee, that feels damn good," he bellows, "try it." I strip to my shorts and jump in as he gets out, soaps up and rinses off under the hose. Alana starts tearing off her clothes, demanding that someone lower her down with a mixture of exuberance and indignation. Mariana hands me the plump little thing and we're inside the dark walls of the well, splashing about in water that is heavenly cool, especially considering that this is the second day the water has been out, and I rode horses in the sun all afternoon before checking out the wrestlers yesterday. It's just what the mad doctor ordered to beat the Mexican heat. Lobo dives in. Our elated voices echo through the dark, cool, cinder-block walls.

Kevin peers over the edge and looks down into the well. "Maricon," he offers as he threatens to spit on us. Just the other night I heard Lobo chant that exact taunt at the wrestlers in Monclova. The wrestling matches were one giant melee of profane insults hurled between the crowd and the "bad guys" in the ring. People's mothers were told to get fucked on a minute-by-minute basis. Toddlers and pre-schoolers sat idly on their parents laps as profanities of every imaginable variety were screamed with comic intensity, flooding down from the bleachers and returned with equal vigor from the performers in the ring. When Lobo saw that many people had brought their kids he expressed regret at leaving Junior with Cassandra. Somewhere between all the insults wrestling did occur: a sloppy, obviously staged brand where the exact formula was duplicated every match, the highlight occurring when the wrestlers would spill into the crowd, smashing each other with the chairs the patrons were just sitting on. The vile brutality of it all was washed away by the endless chorus of jeers and slurs. It was a morbid brand of entertainment, but hooked me and reeled me in.

The whole filthy atmosphere was engaging, almost electric; I just wished I didn't need translations so I could laugh in time with everyone else. Lobo on the other hand found his calling in those rusty bleachers, with all the mean insults flying around him. "Ha. That wrestler just told that fat broad up there to sit her big ass down before he slaps the fat off of it." he rejoiced. The place grew wilder as the night progressed and the beer consumption accumulated. Lobo became nearly possessed by the atmosphere, buckling over in laughter, spewing a drunken, wheezy laugh that seemed on the border of turning into tears at any moment. His low, black voice thundered through the arena constantly, sometimes spontaneously starting mocking chants that rained down upon the wrestlers as the bleachers chimed in behind him.

Back in the well Alana's hoarse laughter fills the concrete walls, and Lobo and I join in. Mariana serenely peers down and soon Kenneth has jumped in too. It's a childish moment, or rather a moment from childhood where the euphoric feeling that you're squeezing all the fun out of an instance that there is to be had sweeps over you and the only important thing is the sound of your laughter. Man, these guys sure know how to laugh, it just flies right out of them. Everyone's having too much fun and Kevin can't resist, a droplet of spit "accidentally" falls from his mouth onto Lobo. In a heartbeat the elder asshole is chasing the younger through the yard. They're both barefoot, but Kevin's feet are used to it, and Lobo soon relents. There's a moment when their dark eyes are glaring at each other and I can see the mutual respect and disdain they have for each other. A timeless second passes until Lobo's son catches his attention and the stare down spell is broken. Junior is on the edge of the porch, pants around his ankles, casually pissing into the grass. "My God," Lobo joyously moans, "we've resorted to savagery of the worst variety." He gleefully clasps his hands as we watch his son finish up his business. La Madrid was seeping into the boy the way it had into his father.

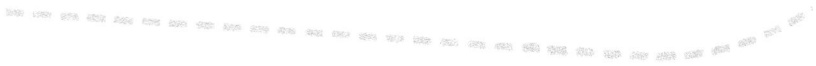

Even One Would Have Been Enough
July 21, 2006

We sped up I-5 in the middle of the night. Originally we had been planning on leaving the apartment we had been renting for the summer around three, but somehow hadn't started until dusk. Lobo, Cassandra, Junior and I crammed the Honda full of tents, sleeping bags, grills, guitars, and our lazy good spirits and headed north for the weekend. The sun cannon-balled into the horizon, splashing orange and gold on the clouds above. Sonny Treadway, an old gospel laptop steel player, blared from the speakers. The sultry rhythms from his groove, along with the golden glow of dusk that flooded in through the windshield, grabbed me and I danced in my seat as we ran.

We had hoped to be at Crater Lake that night, but instead would have to settle for making it to the Oregon line and hitting the lake the next day. Cassandra and Junior slept soundly in the back as I drove and Lobo sat shotgun. The Honda cut through the darkness as we talked over the music. "Man, I can't wait to see the stars in Oregon," I told Lobo. "I can't fucking wait to see how many there are up there in that Oregon sky," I said as I peered up through the windshield.

It was July 2006, about a year before the Honda was stolen at Tubby's—the summer the Honda busted out 17,000 miles without a hitch. I spent a large part of that summer in Chico, California, renting an apartment in the college town and logging six hours a day in a hyperbaric chamber. On weekends I was free to explore California, and that's what we were doing now. Lobo, Cassandra, and Junior had come to stay with me for the last month of the summer. My time spent in the chamber was an attempt to eradicate Lyme disease from my system once and for all. My symptoms weren't even that bad at the time, mostly centering on musculoskeletal pain in my legs, but I was hoping the hyperbaric chamber would be the last step in curing me for good. In truth I would enjoy 18 more months of moderately light symptoms, and one more trek across the continent the following summer, before my body lost further ground to the disease and I had to start nearly from scratch again. Such is life—these are the swings associated with the disease.

The theory behind the chamber was that it simulated the pressure of being deep under water—and being deep under water increased the circulation of blood, which carried the antibiotics to the far recesses of my body. Thus the bacteria would have fewer places to hide. Some people swear by it, but I saw minimal results. There were a lot of really sick people in the chamber with me, most of them with Lyme, though some had other ailments that the increased circulation could help. There was a sixteen-year old girl that the disease had bound to a wheel chair, and she had to be lifted into the chamber each day. She smiled bashfully at us as the nurses struggled to fit her in. There was an old lady with a wound on the side of her head that wouldn't heal. She singled me out one day and told me that all she wanted was to die, that her son had removed all the guns from her home. I didn't know what to tell her. There were funny moments too. Once somebody farted and everyone had to pretend like they didn't smell a thing even though we were all trapped in an airtight container.

Lobo and I swapped stories as Cassandra and Junior slept in the back. "You know they show us movies in the hyperbaric chamber, but what they do is they play the movie on a TV outside the chamber and send the sound in through a speaker. We all watch from a window. The whole capsule is about the size of the back of a van, you understand, real tight. And usually there's like five or six of us in there. Anyways, they had Netflix and each patient would get to pick a movie each day, but I would always pass. You know everyone always picked all these crappy, mainstream movies and I didn't feel like forcing them to watch some indie flick they would think was boring or weird. The first three weeks go on like this, everyday they're like, 'Nick, what movie do you want,' and 'you never pick,' and all that. But I just keep passing. Then I read about a movie called *Keep the River to Your Right* on the back of some book in Borders. I didn't know that much about it. All I knew was that it was about a dude who walked into the Amazon one day, then walked out of it two years later all fucked up. Apparently he had been accepted by some natives in there or something, and seen some intense shit. Pretty tame, right. Well they ask me again, and this movie pops in my head and I tell them to get it for me. It shows up the next day and they start playing it and real quick this movie just goes fucking crazy. This tribe in the Amazon is totally down with homosexuality and cannibalism and this dude had taken a native lover the last time he went in the jungle and eaten humans and the documentary was about him reuniting with the tribe and reuniting with his lover. As the movie goes on all they're talking about is how this whole tribe readily accepts the men fucking each other while raising families with their wives—"

"God bless 'em," added Lobo

"—and how they go out and kill other people and eat them in their spare time. About twenty minutes in everyone keeps giving me these weird, dirty looks, like 'what the hell is wrong with you.' People start inching away from me and shit, like I was trying to decide whether to suck their dick or take a bite out of their leg. Fucking ridiculous. The one movie I pick has to be a documentary about cannibal gays going crazy in the jungle. And I just had to sit there and own up to my movie. Now everyone in that damn chamber was thinking, 'so this is why Nick never requests a movie, because he's a fucking freak—"

"—who's goin' straight to hell," Lobo screamed in laughter as he finished my sentence. "Fuck 'em. Let 'em think what they're gonna think Vittas."

"True."

"That reminds me," he went on, "did I tell you about the fight I got in with Cassandra's mom?" I shook my head. "It was a doozy. Well, she comes in my house, with her bad attitude, spoiling my son when I've specifically told her not to. She disregards me, Vittas. There's only one way to deal with these savages, I swear it. I had enough that day and I told her to get the fuck out of my house, but she wouldn't. So I started grabbing all her shit, her boots, her bag, she was making tamales, I grabbed those out of the oven too, and I threw it all out of the door. I said, 'yo, there's your shit bitch, go get it.' When she did, BANG, I slammed the door in her face. But she's a fiery broad, that one, she wouldn't quit. She was pushing on the door, reaching her hand around. When I grabbed her to throw her out her nails raked my back," he commented with a twisted admiration. "Cassandra's grandmother was there too and I threw her out too, but real gentle, 'cause she is so old." He smiled that evil smile he has when reflecting on any piece of chaos and continued. "Cassandra was screaming at us to stop, and when we wouldn't she went into the closet and closed the door." I laughed behind the wheel until my cheeks hurt.

"Let 'em think what they're gonna think, huh?"

"You know it," he answered with a smile that could light up the darkest cave.

Around midnight we stopped in the town of Ashland, Oregon. Lobo took Cassandra and Junior to our motel room, then asked me if I wanted to go on a walk with him around the parking lot while he smoked a joint. He lit the joint and we walked in the shadows of the streetlights as the sweet smell of marijuana filled the space around him. "You know Nick, I can see how happy you are to be on the road. I saw it when we were driving today, you were beaming with it brother. I knew then that even if there was only one star up in that sky it would have been enough. I just want you to know what a beautiful and powerful thing that is, man." I smiled. "You passed it on to me. When I saw you driving, just so happy, you filled me with something. Life was gleaming through both your eyes Nick." He told me this as his eyes gleamed in the streetlights behind the trailing smoke of the joint that dangled in his mouth and I laughed because he was right, even if I had only seen one star in the sky, that would have been enough.

We went into the motel room but both of us were too charged to sleep. Cassandra and Junior serenely lay on one of the beds and Lobo and I barricaded ourselves in the bathroom and talked for hours into the night. We laughed like lunatics and it seemed that our laughter bounced off the tile walls and grew with each reverberation, like the echo would run on forever in between the bathroom walls. Lobo hunched over on the closed toilet lid, wheezing out his mad laugh as the veins of his throat bulged out like a set of thick ropes straining to hold in an incredibly heavy weight. I brought my guitar in there and lay in the bathtub plucking out tunes when the moment struck me and I needed a break from the laughter.

We traded stories for hours. "This one time I forgot my green card at the border in Mexico and my dad had to drive back and get it for me. He said, 'stay put.' The minute he left I started walking around."

"How old were you?" I asked

"Oh, about twenty. I saw this hole and I started to crawl in it."

"What? What hole?" Often Lobo's stories won't make sense without some heavy questioning on the part of his audience.

"It was a hole in the side of the wall and I crawled right through it. Luckily it was this girl's birthday on the other side. Well, actually it wasn't very lucky. Right when I get through that hole these two guys start walking in stride with me. I was all confidence until one was like 'what ya got?' Man, these border towns are lawless Nick. I started slowly backing away from them, slowly, slowly, and then BANG. I started running for that hole. They chased me and grabbed a hold of me as I was half way through the hole, grabbed my ankle and reached through my pockets. They got my wallet, but it only had a library card in it, and that was expired," Lobo finished as we filled the bathroom with laughter again.

That's the thing about traveling with someone, you have so much time in the car, and motels and campsites that you tell all your stories, you lay them out and piece them together like a giant jigsaw puzzle, and by the time you're done you see your life, your own stories, in a different perspective because you've gone over so many of them in such a short time, and you can see how they link up and fit together like never before.

I couldn't have told you why I needed the road so badly at the time, I just knew that nothing else made me feel as euphoric. The mad stories that filled the car and the mad landscapes that flooded through my eyes all added up to heaven for me. Years later I was asked why I liked to travel so much and the best explanation I could come up with was that there's a balance within you that gets thrown off when you've been sick for years—that years of illness and confinement tilt some scale within you too far in one direction and you have to wander, you have to ramble, to reinstate some form of equilibrium within your soul.

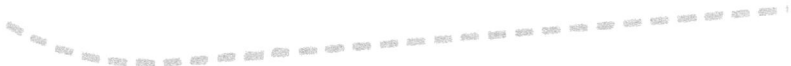

What's In a Bet?
2005–2009

The first bet I ever made was when I was nine years old. I made it with my younger cousin Stavros. It was a fifty-fifty shot as to whether his pregnant mother would have a boy or a girl. My cousin Elena was born several months later and I was out a dollar, which was no chump change back then. Stavros has always been a better gambler than me. Maybe it started even earlier than that. Every New Year's Eve our parents would throw a quarter into the New Year's cake mix before baking it and announce that whoever had the piece with the coin would get five dollars. It was supposed to symbolize good luck for the coming year, but it was a gamble, a lottery with the prospect of easy money making our little hearts thump as the adults doled out each piece in agonizing slow motion. I'd immediately tear through the cake, tracing my tongue through every bite searching for the winning coin. I don't recall ever finding it, but I do remember the smug look of victory Stavros shot me when he bit into that quarter. He must have been all of five years old at the time. Maybe that's when we learned that money won is sweeter than money earned because it comes with adrenaline.

Stavros was the kind of kid that was always scheming to make a buck. When he was in third grade he stole pornos from the seven-eleven and sold them in the bathrooms of his school. He was, and is, a true businessman and has never had any conflicts about making money or taking money. If there was money to be made it was his calling to make it. If there was money to be taken it was his calling to take it. He's a short, cocky runt. Half Greek, half Korean; if you are one who's inclined to believe stereotypes you might say he was bred to gamble. I've never seen him offer anything but a glib sneer at someone who has lost a bet to him. Sympathy isn't even on the radar. He's never scared of losing, he's always charged by the prospect of winning, and the notion that he can take it from someone else offers a near intoxication for him. Since graduating from college he's lived in Atlantic City, Las Vegas, and Los Angeles; all of which offer the lure of legalized gambling or at the very least legalized poker.

I started playing poker with my high school friends, and really began to devote serious time to the endeavor once I was forced to give up basketball for the second time in 2005. It was then that I began playing with Stavros and I started betting and making, what was for me, real money. He lived in Atlantic City at the time and had some kind of entry-level position in the Tropicana casino. Once a month or so I'd drive up from DC on the weekends and partake in the long, marathon sessions at the card tables that were a regular habit for him. A typical weekend went something like: arrive at Atlantic City on a Friday night, eat a hurried dinner, head down to the poker tables and grind it out until some point into Saturday. I'd usually quit after 12-15 hours and stumble back to his apartment in a delirious haze. After a poker session my mind was exhausted, but also stuck in this high gear of stress and analytical thinking. This was due to the cutthroat rhythm of constantly hunting the people sitting with me at the table while conscious that they're laying traps for my chips too. To relax is to lose. I'd pull the curtains shut and try to sleep only to realize that the nervous energy of the tables had followed me home and, even though I was dog tired, the thoughts in my head were still moving at the fast pace and intense weight of the game. Stavros's endurance far out matched mine. I usually wouldn't see him until Saturday night, where he'd come home for two or three hours of what had to be restless sleep, then attack the poker room again, usually playing straight through Sunday. I'd join him on Saturday night, play through until Sunday morning, then drive home after a short nap in his apartment.

Often I questioned why I had adopted a hobby that contradicted my core belief that greed is a sinful, limiting emotion that is the crux of many individuals and society as a whole. How odd it was that as someone who considered himself a bleeding liberal, a near socialist, would devote so much time to such a capitalist endeavor. How odd it was that I, someone who meditated daily, practiced yoga, and focused earnest attention on his spiritual evolution, was completely enveloped into the gains and losses of poker. But then again I've always been attracted to the rush of the gamble and told myself it was one way to assert that money had no power over me because I so gladly risked it. There is some truth to this because a good gambler can't have a strong attachment to his money, but it's a half-truth at best. The power of gambling is fulfilling a greedy impulse and there's no way around that fact. But this was hard to see when I was riding a hot winning streak.

My eyes often burned in exhaustion on the three-hour trip home from AC to DC, but I rode the high that the warm glow of money stuffed in my pocket gave me all the way down I-95. I replayed winning hands over in my mind and relived the euphoric sensation of raking in chips and feeling like I had it all figured out. I can't lie, it was sweet to think that I had out smarted someone and ran off with a nice profit for my conquest.

Poker is actually more of a skill than a gamble. Because I'm pitted against fellow players I don't have to face the weighted odds of betting against the house like I would in black jack or craps. But there's definitely a gamble to poker as well. The skill comes in placing myself with a 65-80% chance of winning a hand before the remaining cards are dealt. The skill comes in reading the players around me, analyzing their betting patterns, breaking down each aspect of the hand as it transpires and finding the clues that tell me what their cards are. There are clues everywhere, but you've got to pay attention. It's a meticulous practice that takes an intense dedication to withstand over the course of a 15-hour session. And after all this, even if I play a hand perfectly, I still have to gamble, though the gamble is heavily weighted in my favor. If I get someone to move all in at the start of a hand with pocket Jacks and I've got Aces, I'm a four to one favorite to win. That being said, 20% of the time I'll lose. And here is where the most important skill comes into play. The game is so stressful and full of so many traps that everyone at the table is setting for me, that when I do play a hand perfectly and still lose a disgust for the cruelty of the game builds up within me. At times I can sift through hours of dead cards until finally coming across a ripe opportunity, play it to perfection and still lose. That's the loss that is bitter. If that scene is repeated several times over the course of the night, the bitterness can brew and erupt into being "on tilt".

Being on tilt is a senseless, petulant emotion that sweeps over people and drives them to rebel against the sensibilities of poker. The word fits the emotion. When I'm on tilt I literally feel like I've slipped off the edge of rationality. Odds mean nothing to me. I could know that an opponent has 70% chance of winning a hand and I still can't wait to throw every last chip into the pot. It's an act of defiance against this ridiculous, strenuous game I've devoted so much time and energy to. It's an act of desperation, trying anything other than the calm, patient route because there's always a chance of winning with enough luck. There are hints of self-loathing for placing myself in this pressurized situation to begin with and the oddly gratifying sensation of watching all my money vanish in a matter of minutes because I'm disgusted with the pursuit of it. It's a very complex thing. Regardless, after the basics of poker, suppressing the urge to go on tilt is the most important and exhausting skill a poker player must apply.

I guess the great cycle of gains and losses that defined my poker career started once I began playing in Atlantic City. It was there that I honed the art of suppressing the urge to go on tilt. I was never the most gifted player. Mine was a standard, conservative style of poker, mostly playing strong cards in safe situations and throwing in an occasional bluff so as not to be too predictable. I would do my best to avoid strong players and prey on weaker ones. And if anyone was clearly on tilt I leapt at the chance to take advantage of them and gleefully scooped up the chips they were hemorrhaging. Stavros was much more dynamic, and subsequently enjoyed much larger profits than I did. I set an hourly rate of 40 dollars an hour as a goal and met it over the course of three months.

On occasion I'd stop for a moment and really observe the tensely wound players around me, the ones that weren't drunk one-timers, content to sit down and flush away a couple of hundred bucks because poker is as good a way to gamble as roulette or craps. At best these regulars had a nervous, sly part to their mouths, and an anxious craving in their eyes; at worst they were crippled, mangled shells of men, wound so tightly by the burden of their compulsion that I could almost see them tearing at the seams. I knew I felt the way those haggard men of the latter group looked on many an instance, but not seeing myself that way allowed me to dismiss it as part of the process that poker demands. And the sly mouthed predator in me won often enough that I avoided looking directly at mirrors at the end of the night and kept coming back.

As the summer of 2006 approached I had built a nice bankroll of 2,700 bucks. Even after all my pre-trip expenses I had a thick wad of 2,300 dollars in cash to play around with on the road. Add this to the fact that my buddy Jack and I were planning on spending the summer in California, (and all its poker rooms), and I assumed there was a great chance that I would return from a three month vacation richer than when I left.

Those aspirations died on our first night in Lake Tahoe. We were both amped for a run in the casinos and decided to enjoy a hike through the mountains during the day to balance out the indulgence of our degenerative behaviors that awaited us at the tables. During the hike the zipper on my backpack loosened and my backpack flipped open. I probably walked several hundred yards before realizing it. I zipped it up and kept going, thinking nothing of it until arriving at the casino that night. At the cashier's window I reached into the backpack to pull out my bankroll and felt nothing. A twinge of panic fluttered through me as I started to frantically grope every corner of every pocket. I did everything to deny what I knew for a fact: I had dropped 2,300 dollars on a trail. I had dropped 2,300 dollars, wrapped in a neat bundle with a rubber band, on the trail. It was unbelievable and I didn't fully accept the fact that the money was gone, that all those grueling hours at the tables were wasted, until I walked down the infamous trail again, scouring every inch for a big bundle of cash. Some hiker had inevitably experienced a religious conversion upon finding a couple grand gift-wrapped for him. Don't ask me why I carried the money with me. I have no idea. The loss of the money was bad, but the wasted effort in Atlantic City was what really bothered me. By dropping that money I squandered sixty hours of suppressing tilt, sixty hours of battling against the sinister intentions of a table full of players who were scheming for my chips while my mind ran on overdrive to scam for theirs. Sixty hours engulfed by the pursuit of easy money and all the subsequent emotional roller coasters that come along. Sixty hours I could have devoted to anything more productive than the cultivation and realization of greed. I came to see that I didn't really like playing cards, I liked winning at cards. There's a big difference. How beneficial can an activity be that I only enjoy when I win? That wasn't the case with other competitive endeavors I partook in. Win or lose, I always loved basketball and had an intense gratitude for the privilege to play every time I stepped on the court. Comparatively I would straight curse the tables after a losing night. With that correlation I decided to give up poker altogether. For the rest of the trip I left Jack at the poker rooms around California and heard about his conquests or devastating defeats the next day. And this suited me fine, though my funds almost ran dry before I returned home.

The day I returned home Stavros called me and asked me if I wanted to hit this lush home game he had discovered deep in the suburbs of DC. "It's at this dentist's house in Potomac, and he's a maniac. I couldn't believe the things this guy was doing," Stavros chuckled. I could hear the cash register ringing in his mind. "I've never seen anyone go on tilt like this guy. All the tells were there, nostrils flaring, everything. For a while I thought he was doing coke in the bathroom, but I think he just can't control his betting. He had the whole table going crazy. It's the perfect game." It was a convincing argument. I had 140 dollars to my name. I went upstairs and secretly borrowed another hundred from my mother's nightstand, deciding to give the game one more chance. Had I lost all the money that night my poker career would have been over.

The parking lot outside the dentist's office was filled with BMWs, Mercedes, and Audis. My dented old Honda stood out, just like I stood out around all the well-dressed playboys inside. I walked into Farouk "the dentist" Adnan's game, which he held in the basement under his office, and instantly knew I'd walked into a goldmine. He was a handsome, well-groomed Arab, slender with a cocky air about him. The whole table gravitated around his personality and he obviously loved the attention. In a game where you're involved in a big hand several times a night, he was wrapped up in three huge hands within the first half hour. Farouk was an action junkie and his chip stack wildly fluctuated reflecting his erratic play. He refused to budge off of any pot and made ridiculous, stupid calls making sure that no one could bluff him, even if it cost him hundreds of dollars. On the other hand he made wild stabs at pots, gloating mercilessly when a bluff paid off. "I got nothing," he moaned joyously, turning his cards over for the table to see. "How do you fold there, man? You folded top pair and I had nothing." He was the picture of a sore winner. And when his bluffs were called he steamed and reloaded, throwing another 200, 300, or 500 into the bank for a new set of chips. I've never seen anyone burn through money like he did. He didn't always lose big though, many times he won big too. That's what the nature of his play demands, big gains and bigger losses. Over the course of four months I saw him lose anywhere from 1,000-1,500 dollars on many nights, but I also saw him crush the game when he got on a hot streak for 3,000 dollars, which is no easy feat at 1-2, or 2-4 no limit. Of course he never broke even. His wild style affected the whole table and chips were flying back and forth at a frantic pace. I struggled not to get caught up in it and bided my time, waiting for choice opportunities to pick off someone's mistake.

I sat quietly and played tightly, trying earnestly to play hands with Farouk heads up. I had just re-read *One Flew Over the Cuckoo's Nest* on the ride home and I started to channel the spirit of Randle McMurphy, the smooth talking gambler from the novel. I saw the hustle laid out in front of me and snatched it. When I talked, I almost felt like McMurphy was whispering the words in my ear before I said them. I wanted the dentist to like me and think that he had won my respect. Most of all I wanted him to keep playing his woeful brand of reckless poker. "That was a strong bet man, it could have worked really differently," I muttered as he dumped off 90 dollars in chips with an obvious bluff. On the next bluff that blew up in his face I casually mentioned, "you put him to the test though," as I dealt out the cards. When his careless play paid off I made sure to compliment that. Always quietly, so he barely heard, as if I was talking to myself, "man, I couldn't make that move," like I was envious. When I beat him I would immediately claim it was luck, putting on an air that I was glad to have escaped him. Stavros was doing the same thing. I tried not to be obvious while feeding the notion that I feared him because I saw that along with the adrenaline of the gamble, that was what he coveted most, to be feared and respected. I made 600 dollars on my first night and barely broke a sweat. It was easy money. When I noticed how agitated Farouk got when his buddy left a five-dollar tip after winning 1,100 dollars I left 50. I was going to do all I could to stay in this game.

I became a regular at his game and the conversational dance between the two of us continued. Picking him off became a sport to me. After studying him for a while I knew when he had it and when he didn't, how to incite a call on not only the hand we were involved in but the next one too. I learned exactly what amount of money got his adrenaline pumping, and how much to bet to coax him into trying to bluff me out of a pot I knew for a fact I had the best hand in. At times I'd feel guilty about manipulating him so mercilessly. I rationalized it by citing that manipulation was the nature of the game and, if he could, Farouk would gleefully clean me out in a heartbeat. I told myself that a cutthroat mentality is by definition the foundation of poker. Stavros told me this too and I listened. "You're not forcing him to play that way. He's got a style of play that lends itself to big wins or big losses." The undertone was that if Farouk was going to wield his money around like a weapon it was only fair to turn that weapon against him. There's some truth to this view, but what about not playing altogether? The latter option was completely implausible to Stavros and I left it out of our debate. The rationalization became a little harder to justify after I found out that he had a real gambling problem. Apparently poker was just child's play, and like many addicts, he'd fallen in love with sports betting. Stavros told me that Farouk was attending Gamblers' Anonymous meetings, but was spiraling so wildly out of control that he was calling in bets from the meetings. When I heard this I became pretty torn about the whole thing, though not torn enough to stop going to his game every couple of weeks. Later on I heard that his gambling was causing marital problems and I became keenly aware that the hustle had lured me again.

Before working in a pre-school I had been a manager in a used CD store/pawn shop for five years. My job was to hustle people for their CDs, DVDs, stereos, etc. I had to gauge the lowest amount of money I could offer for their stuff and still have them return to sell me more in the future. If they were selling a whole mass of CDs and movies I knew they were desperate and took advantage, offering less because I knew they eventually had to take the money. Their return business didn't matter because they had sold pretty much all they had anyways. There was no room for empathy in that business and I became adept at sizing up exactly what something was worth to someone, then offering a little less. I did other things in that job that I'm not proud of too. I openly encouraged neighborhood kids to steal from Best Buy or Wal-Mart. I would buy 15 copies of the newest DVD, sealed in plastic, from the same group of thugs on a bi-weekly basis. When one group got busted a new one would step right in its place. We got to the point where kids were asking me what movies I wanted and coming back the next day with bags of freshly shoplifted copies. None of this really sat well with me, but again I rationalized that this was the job I had and this was the society I lived in. When I went to the car dealer they tried (and succeeded) in selling me parts I didn't need and I understood that it wasn't personal, that the mechanics had bosses breathing down their necks just like me, and had to produce numbers just like I did. And so we were all participants in the great dance of exploitation, the hustle, be hustled two-step of monetary exchange. But when I quit that job to work in the pre-school I thought I'd left my end of the scheming behind, but apparently it was harder to shed than I'd originally thought. Somehow the hustle followed me.

Farouk stopped calling me after four months. The only time I ever lost money was the last time I went to his house, almost like he was waiting for me to lose one time and then boot me out of his game. No matter, by that point I'd built a healthy bankroll of 2,500 dollars. When I came home from Farouk's, usually as dawn was rearing a reproachful eye, I would lie on my mattress with a smirk glued to my face. There is a slice of Stavros in me. I can't deny that I loved beating people; I loved competing and coming home with the tangible trophy of 500 dollars for my efforts. I'd like to say there was a great conflict within me as to whether I should be devoting so much time and energy to swindling people within the framework of a set of rules, but there wasn't. The pursuit of easy money mixed with the charging narcotic of competition was an irresistible lure and I quickly found the next game to attack.

I heard about an underground card room down by the Capital off Pennsylvania Avenue. This Ivy league bull named Jared ran it. He was imposing in both stature and character and held an iron fist of discipline over the action that I've never seen matched at any legitimate casino. The game was held over a restaurant. The entrance was behind a slender, dark, back alley, enclosed by three sets of towering apartment buildings and the restaurant on the far end. Rats scurried from overflowing dumpsters, and occasionally I stepped over a fresh batch of pink vomit on my way to the long metal staircase that led to a rusted, iron door. Cameras peered down from multiple angles. The whole atmosphere was slightly intimidating. Inside dealers sat at the tables that you were supposed to tip just like in a casino. A fridge stocked with drinks sat by the filthy bathroom and a couple of flat screens stood mounted on the walls. The level of play was much better at Jared's than at Farouk's. On any given night there were at least four players that I tried to avoid getting tangled up with. This place wasn't a friendly home game. The sour faced, foul-mouthed, dregs of society were attracted to a place like Jared's. They were not out to have fun, they were out to make money and subsequently a palpable intensity blanketed every corner of the poker room.

The characters, who willingly or begrudgingly, love a place like Jared's are unique in their grimy, desperate way. They offer their own form of reality TV by polluting it with their populace. There was Benny, the 27 year-old drunk that stumbled in at 2:30 in the morning. After berating an opponent for an excruciatingly long time Jared decided that Benny was too drunk to play that night. "What?" Benny proclaimed, "I'm not too drunk to play, look at how many cards I'm folding." He was probably right too, though he was loud and gregariously ball busting everyone around him with a slew of disgusting, curse laden, sexual jokes. Benny was a true animal and the shinning jewel of a poker room like this. He was like a standup comic that could rob me blind if I wasn't careful. Jared let him off with a stern warning, to which Benny muttered, "I'll give your mother a firm warning."

Next to Benny sat Charlie, the sad faced, stocky Syrian. He scratched his baldhead every several minutes and muttered,

"Oh, God. I have to be at work tomorrow. Tomorrow morning at seven I gotta go to work." He repeated this until Benny finally popped off at him, "Charlie, you fucking moron it's six o'clock. Tomorrow is today, man." Charlie hung his head at the devastating news that the day had reached him within this filthy pit again. His meek eyes darted around at the chip stacks of those next to him, and back down at his, that used to be up to 700, but now was teetering around 150. He complained about minor infractions that had cost him, but in a weak way that invited the Ivy league bully who ran the place to make an example out of him and give him a time out. Jared forced Charlie to walk all the way across to the other side of the room as the rest of the table laughed. Charlie complained from the corner, but he didn't dare cross the line that Jared had set for him. He was somewhat of a whipping boy, but everyone loved him for it.

Lamar, the 30 year-old light skinned brother, sat next to Charlie's spot. He was long and lanky and always had a boyish grin smirking on his face. Lamar casually sipped at a single bourbon on the rocks all night and made one goofy joke after another. He was too cool and calm to be put on edge by the grinding pressure of the room and I tried to stay out of his way. Chris, a behemoth 300-pound whale of a man, and Jake, possibly even bigger, sat at opposite ends of the table with opposite styles of play. Chris was loose and crazy, prepared to lose 1,000 dollars on any hand just for the chance to feel the rush of the gamble. Jake was tight and patient, content to sit night in and night out grind out a hard way to make an easy living. Jake has been doing this for decades and I wanted no part of him. They looked so similar I might mistake one for the other if not for the seesawing chip stack that rose and fell in front of Chris. In between them was Rob, a classic internet poker punk, drunk on too many poker shows, convinced that he was one step away from becoming the game's next superstar and intent on telling anyone and everyone how poorly they played. And then there was me, quiet, unassuming, my game was in the mold of Jake's, though not as adept as his because he had years of experience to draw on when trying to get a good read on a player.

And it was there, with these people that I chose to spend many a night, far past the night and into the coming morning actually. In that grimy room my leg constantly jittered, no matter how tired I was, because I was caught in a gambling arena and all of us knew that gambling creates an unseen, electric energy that sweeps over a room. We were all charged with the weary eyed intoxication that winning money gave us and we were all unspoken brethren in the quest for this high. We were all trying to take it from one another.

Money ruled the night. Money consumed my every thought and action for hours on end. Money. *How much do I have, how much have I made so far?* Money. *How can I get his chips, how is he trying to steal mine?* Money. *If I fold here am I throwing money away like a coward or cutting my losses like a seasoned pro?* Money. *Freeze your face like a statue, Nick, before he figures out you got nothing.*

Money, the invisible drug, a sniff of it sets a rush of adrenaline careening through my veins. By five o'clock in the morning I hadn't won a hand in hours and the night was slipping away into futility. I had battled all night against a parade of worthless cards, deliberately climbing out of a 300-dollar hole that I fell into in the first hours until I was back to even again. I hadn't said a word in hours. I didn't have the energy. My eyes burned with exhaustion and I was beginning to curse myself for coming and devoting yet another night to these degenerates. I was dealt a pocket pair of nines. First decent hand I'd seen in three hours. Rob, the internet-punk, raised my 40-dollar bet on the flop to 120. I had my pocket nines, an over pair to the board and the range of hands he could have ran through my mind as if on a treadmill. *Has he hit a set, in which case I'd basically be drawing dead? Does he have a higher over pair? Why wouldn't he have raised me before the flop? Could this be a trap? Maybe he has a draw; there are two clubs on the board?* All these options and many more swam around my head like a school of fish gasping for air in a puddle. Something didn't feel right. I went with my gut and re-raised him all in and Rob instantly called me. He didn't even think about it, and I was sure my night was over, but it turned out he had a gut-shot and a flush draw. We were basically staging a coin flip for 720 dollars. My heart was beating so wildly I could feel the blood surging through my body, running up the sides of my temples like a set of rapids, flooding my brain. The cards were dealt before I could process them and the dealer was sliding a huge mound of chips toward me when I realized I had won. A euphoric sigh of relief leaked out of me, more of an involuntary decompression that had a full body effect as all the tension that had built up over the hand ran up the pathways of my sternum and escaped from my nostrils. An impromptu enthusiasm for life infected me. The win charged my tongue with the uncontrollable urge to babble something, anything. I was juiced and they all knew it. "Look whose ready to chat all of a sudden, " Chris snorted. He knew that winning is the drug. One more big hand in the next hour and I was up a cool thousand. I cashed out a little before six. I put 500 in one sock and 500 in the other, three hundred in my pocket and said a silent prayer that no one in the room had texted their boy to meet me in the alley. I floated on out of the place like I had just punched my time card. The iron door clanged shut behind me and I scampered down the metal staircase, then leapt into an all out sprint down the dark streets of DC with a thousand dollars in my socks and the airy feeling of victory in my chest. The cold, night air tasted like chilled wine pumping through my lungs. I got to my car, jumped into the driver's seat and sped off, giddy with the prospect of getting home and counting all that money. When I got home I counted and re-counted that bundle of cash. Each time my fingers traced over the bills I got a shot of the wonderful, triumphant feeling that scooping up Rob's chips gave me hours before. The afterglow of winning drifted into the next day, touching every moment I walked through. Even the fatigue that dragged behind me like an anchor on land kicked up wistful feelings of victory. And this is how I would feel after a winning night.

A completely opposite sensation would engulf me on losing nights. There's no walk lonelier than a loser's. Sick with the realization that I'd spent ten hours surrounded by degenerate crooks that had wanted nothing else other than to swindle me, I almost welcomed the prospect of being held up because it would give me the opportunity to tell my muggers they had missed their chance, all my money had been left on the table. All the grimy charm of the characters at Jared's was washed away when I'd lose. I just saw them as blathering mouths of revulsion, and the night turned into a mocking mirror of my greed, and the inevitable exhaustion of the following day simply served to remind me of the depths that my gluttonous soul could drag me to. I'd wonder why I put myself through such a thing, but the answer was simple enough; more often than not I won. As the summer of 2007 approached I had a nice bankroll of over 5,000 dollars saved up. Determined to avoid last year's fiasco, I deposited the money in the bank and left with Jack and Costa for the West coast again.

The trip ran straight into a brick wall in Oakland, where my car was stolen. On top of that the car had been packed to the brim with all the camping equipment, cameras, guitars and the like that one would take on a ninety day journey. Add the cost of replacing three months worth of meds and even though I ended up retrieving the vehicle five weeks later I still lost close to 5,000 dollars worth of stuff. How's that for symmetry. Sitting on the front porch steps of Costa's uncle's friend's house, staring at the empty parking spot that used to house my beloved Honda, it dawned on me that all those countless hours spent scheming for money had somehow cultivated this. It's too simple to say, "You reap what you sow," because obviously many people make a living conniving for a buck and don't suffer any symmetrical losses. If Stavros was to reap what he sowed for all the hours he hustled at the tables, he may be in debt for the rest of his life, but he won't. He's a gambler and a winner, and that's all there is to it. Maybe it was the conflict within me, the one that I always ignored or pushed aside to enjoy the intoxication of the gamble, maybe that internal conflict somehow shot back all the energy and effort I focused on taking other people's money into a rain of financial losses on me. I'd never felt completely at ease with the cutthroat, gluttony of poker, (though obviously I was comfortable enough to allow myself to be lured back again and again), and perhaps this disharmony of money lust and repulsion for the brutish materialism at the core of the game set in motion a course of events that always ended with me losing the money I'd won. So, was I setting myself up to lose my winnings because I didn't feel right about how I'd attained them? Was there some greater internal force beyond the constraints of my personal ego that was trying to alter the focus of my free time, which somehow read the road maps of the brewing future and led me down the specific paths that ended with the loss of money won? Was there some Karmic aspect demanding that all the insatiable, craving energy I projected out into the universe was duplicated and sent right back to me? I didn't know, but as I sat on those steps the loss of my car seemed to funnel back to the clear sensation that I had been wasting my time at the poker tables, regardless of the outcome.

And with that realization my poker career began it's slow decent into retirement. When I came home I played in occasional home games with my friends, or entered a tournament that Stavros would host if he were visiting town, but I didn't seek out games like Farouk's or Jared's. I no longer saw poker as a worthy dedication of time and effort. I no longer saw poker as a necessary way to supplement my income. I stopped keeping spreadsheets marking my nightly progress at the tables.

Two years later I found myself stranded in Kalispell, Montana. I'd moved to Texas and Jack and I had taken the RV I was living in on a road trip instead of the trusted, dependable Honda. Big mistake. We blew through the rear four tires because the rig had a bent housing axle and were caught waiting for the new set of tires to be delivered from the next town over. Across the street from the motel we were staying in hung the glowing neon sign for the Cattleman Casino, the softest game I've ever had the pleasure of encountering. It was a 2-5 no limit game, with a 300 dollar maximum pot, which entices the awful players to play even worse because the most they can lose in one hand is 150 dollars. The one room casino was nothing more than an addition to the bar and was filled with gentle, mild mannered locals that seemed to enjoy a friendly game of cards between each other on a nightly basis. Jack and I were nothing short of sharks in a place like that. I toyed with grandmothers that may as well have broadcast their weak hands with a megaphone, begging me to steamroll them with a strong bluff, to which I gleefully obliged. All the old instincts kicked in with one, strong, over powering, salivating breath. I picked off absurd, senselessly aggressive bluffs from the men who wanted to put me in my place and then strung them along to squeeze the maximum out of them when I hit a hand. It was so easy I felt open pangs of guilt for taking such merciless advantage of their clueless, infantile understanding of poker. But I couldn't stop myself. My Chip stack grew as if it was on steroids, until I was sitting on 1,200 dollars by the time the game shut down at three in the morning. Ha. What an early night. I sauntered out into the Montana night with 1,000 fresh dollars in my pocket. The cool, dewy breeze hit the greedy, shit-eating grin of a shameless capitalist as I snickered all the way back to my room.

I stopped by Nashville on the way back to Austin. The Cattleman Casino had paid for the new tires and left 400 dollars to spare. I'd wanted to check out the music scene in Nashville and it didn't disappoint. Only thing was that I had to park the RV off the beaten path because it's hard to park that thing in a city. As I approached the RV a car pulled up and this black dude leaned out of the window. There was a woman sitting next to him. "You know where the Knight's Inn is at?" he hollered at me with a big grin. I told him I didn't as the car cruised up to me. He stepped out of his car, took a quick glance around the deserted back street and instantly his whole demeanor changed. His shoulders hunched forward and he lumbered toward me as he reached behind his back at his waistband. *Well, this can't be good*, I thought to myself right before he glowered, "give me all your fucking money."

"Are you serious?" I moaned more to the sky than him. I knew he was very serious.

"Give me all your money or I will kill you," he screamed, clutching at the back of his waist frantically. His girlfriend sat silently in the car and self-consciously painted her nails with a look of agonizing boredom on her face. He probably didn't have a gun, but I didn't want to fight him either and knew I would have had to if I protested. I was cornered on the passenger side of the RV, with the keys dangling in the kitchen door and this man heaving desperate breaths on me.

"Can I just keep my cards, man?" I asked him as I ran over the horrible mental inventory of all the IDs and debit cards I'd have to reissue.

"Just give me the damn money." *Sweet.* I thought to myself, *best mugger ever.* I dug into my pocket to hand over my money like I'd just won a game show. Basically all you have to do is aggressively ask me for money and I'll give it to you.

"It's your lucky fucking day," I told him with a laugh as I handed him the rest of the Cattleman winnings. His eyes bulged at the wad. He snatched the money and leapt back into his car. As he sped off he screamed, "Nashville don't play."

I laughed all the way to Austin. I felt like the universe was sending me a muffled message through a wall. I could hear the rhythm and the tone. I could make a general sketch of what I was being told, but the specifics were lost in a murmur of bass and treble. Just like when you're in one room and can't make out exactly what's being said in the next. I couldn't clearly see the specific reason why some force seemed to be stealing from me the way I stole from others, though I thought I had a sense of it. Like I said before, I'm inclined to believe the internal conflict over the gross materialism implicit in the game and my overall aversion to such a capitalistic outlook outside of the poker tables played a major role. Just how I'm not sure. I'm not saying being an entrepreneur is a spiritually devoid thing, because it's not my place to make that judgment, and things are rarely black or white anyway; just that perhaps in my individual case my spiritual evolution was served by leaving the hustle behind. At the very least the bizarre string of losses attached to poker wins made a strong case to leave my gambling days in the past and I listened, though it isn't always easy to. To this day the betting instinct is strong in me. Jack or Costa will say some stupid thing about basketball and the first words to fly out of my mouth are, "bet me." I watch poker shows on TV and my heart races as they deal the flop. I can't help but imagine that I'm playing the hand, analyzing what I would do if I was sitting at the table, and I get a little vicarious rush. For now that's enough.

Invisibly Ill

I am Invisibly ill. I look healthy. For all intents and purposes I appear today, and have appeared throughout all 14 years of my illness, to be an average young man. I don't walk with a limp, sit in a wheelchair, or have my daily movements impaired by some noticeable neurological disorder; and this fact, no doubt, is a blessing, but a blessing that comes with its own set of challenges. Appearing healthy and being healthy are two different things. An invisible illness can breed a lot of misunderstanding between you and the world around you. When people see you as a seemingly healthy young man they subconsciously place a set of expectations upon you. But, if you happen to be sick in a way that isn't obvious, those expectations can become another burden to carry on top of an already heavy load.

Early on in my illness people's perception of my condition bothered me greatly. I was highly competitive and put a lot of stake in being strong, both physically and mentally. I worked out incessantly, which covered the physical part, but also took pride in exerting my will on social settings, on being one of the madmen on center stage. All that vanished instantly in December of 1997, when I got that first headache doing pushups. Sports and exercise were out of the question, but so was expending the energy to be a fun loving, wild 20-year old. This loss was hard, and for a while I was kind of left without an identity, but what was equally difficult was the suspicion that my friends didn't see the extent that my bodily pains limited me.

A month after moving back to DC from Umass in the winter of 1998, my cousin Stavros and I went to Costa's house. I'd given up on drinking because when I got drunk I pretended nothing was wrong with my body, acted as wild and crazy as I could, then paid for it horribly for weeks afterwards. Weed was still part of my daily routine though, and the three of us smoked a joint next to the ping-pong table in the basement. As the high kicked in Costa picked up one of the paddles and raised an eyebrow in challenge. Stavros jumped on it, "five dollars a game," he proclaimed and the two of them went at it. I wanted to play badly, but had reservations as well. My neck and back hurt already, how would I be able to keep hanging out with them if I played and made it worse? What would I do if the pain became unmanageable? Would I lie down right there in front of them? Would they think I was soft, a drama queen?

Costa won and it was my turn. I grabbed the paddle and the initial exhilaration of the competition, and the accompanying adrenaline rush, masked the pain. I started out a little tentative, but midway through the game I was cutting back and forth, wailing away at the ball with all my might. I won my first two games, and talked a lot of shit doing it. But by the middle of the second game I could feel my back seizing up. I played the last few points gingerly, but still managed to win. The third game was a mistake, but I didn't want to appear to be making excuses for myself. My back locked up, I could barely move. I stood motionless and tried to reach for the ball as tenderly as possible. I got blown out. My night should have ended there, though Stavros and Costa pressured me to play the winner of their game, and laughed when I got blown out again. As Costa drove me home, a bitterness filled me. They didn't understand. They thought my back hurt, so I couldn't play basketball and never equated the limitations of my pain to something as mild as ping-pong. They thought they were better than me, and childishly this wounded my pride. They laughed and talked shit all the way to my house as I tried to smile through the stabbing pain in my back. I guess it wasn't their fault, they were 18 and 20-year old kids, how could they know what back pain felt like?

I went down to my room in my parents' basement completely devastated. I lay down on the floor with my back locked up in agony and stared up at the ceiling, wondering what had happened to my youth. I wanted Costa and Stavros to know what the pain did to me without having to tell them, because I didn't want to come across as a whiner. Aside from that, the truth was too hard for me to hear myself say, I was a 20-year with neck and back pain severe enough to make playing ping pong an impossibility. Worst of all, at that time, I had no diagnosis, and therefore lacked an explanation for my symptoms to, not only myself, but my friends as well.

With my diagnosis in October of 2000 at least I had something I could point to as the cause of my symptoms. But people still have a tendency to forget when they can't see them. I frequently have to balance what friends ask me to do with what the disease demands of me. For example, if I'm hanging out with a friend and a particularly bad headache emerges, that friend will have to be really adept at reading me to understand that I can't stay up late and talk to him because of the symptom, not because I've lost interest or am generally apathetic.

And there's still the question about how much to disclose to people. Will they think I'm complaining or whining? This comes up at work a lot. I've been working in preschools for the past seven years. As one of the few, or only males, on staff I'm often asked to lift or move things that are beyond my means. My co-workers can't see my inflamed back or tight neck, all they see is a man in a school full of women who should help move this table or that shelf. And so I've found ways to allude to my symptoms without getting into the details of the disease because I don't want to be that guy who complains all the time. The invisible nature of the disease forces me to navigate through social situations like these. It just happens to be that when I'm feeling the worst I have to deal with this added burden the most.

Two-Month Experiment
July–October 2000

"Those that make you return, for whatever reason,
to God's solitude, be grateful to them. Worry about the others,
who give you delicious comforts that keep you away from prayer."
—Rumi

Eleven years ago I had a real bleak outlook. I had dropped out of Umass three years prior after I felt a pop in my head during one of my workouts and everything turned white. When I came to I felt like a zombie and immediately went to sleep for several hours. That may have been my first seizure and marked the beginning of a steady decline in which pain spread throughout my body to the point where I could barely walk, and even in sleep I was haunted by dreams of aching muscles. In the most vivid, recurring dream I found myself in the subway station as a train I needed to board pulled up. The train was right there, but my legs throbbed so badly I couldn't stand, and as I crawled toward the car, the doors would shut and the train would race off. I was helpless as the light from the receding train faded into the tunnel. The craziest thing was that the pain was just as real in sleep as it was when I was awake. The bottom of that decline ended on July 27th, 2000 when I crashed into a legit seizure. I was walking through my kitchen to the living room when I started feeling light headed. Then the periphery of my vision started to turn white in constricting circles until I couldn't see. When I woke up I was lying on the floor. The back of my head rang sharply as I lay in a puddle of my own urine. In those years a new part of my body broke down and stayed broke down every six months, starting with my neck, then my back, my hands, and finally my legs. So there was a real fear that this was just the way things were going to be from then on; that I may have to walk in fear of random seizures on top of everything else. I remember lying on the couch in the basement and a well of anger erupted in me. I started thrashing about, beating the pillows. I used to be an athlete. I used to be a fucking maniac. Now I was nothing but a geriatric twenty two year old. I screamed, "What do you want from me." I don't really know whom I was screaming at and right after my body ached twice as bad as a result of my little tantrum.

My mother carried me in the following weeks and I don't know how deep a pit of depression I would have fallen into if not for her. She drove me to Great Falls State Park almost every day and we'd slowly walk five minutes from the parking lot to the overpass looking down on the rapids. That was about all the exertion I could handle. She'd tell me that she knew things were going to work out and for some reason her words had an effect on me. I didn't believe her exactly, but she managed to calm the anxious panic that consumed me since the seizure. I began to look forward to those trips, even structured my hours of emptiness around the prospect of getting out there. But still, I wasn't really living, I was just holding on.

I held on until a couple of months later when I came upon a book that convinced me to give faith a try. It doesn't really matter what book it was because I went back and reread it several years later and found it to be naïve and completely lacking the magic I swore it had in the past, it was just what I needed to hear at that time. The book put the idea in my head that there was a benevolent force beyond myself that could aid me if I offered it a bridge to reach me. That bridge was faith. The concept was simple enough but I was still uneasy about the whole thing. I almost felt selfish asking for help when so many others were enduring so much more. For years I'd structured my spiritual beliefs around the notion that there was a creative force in the universe, but that this force just continued to churn out reality, impartially witnessing the consciousness it created. In many ways I felt like we were on our own after our conception, that our existence was all our creator was invested in. So you see, it was a great contradiction to suddenly start believing that God cared for me only when I needed It the most. There was also the fear of letting my guard down, of being crushed by disappointment when my health remained the same, or got worse. But I took an inventory of my life. I was desperately lonely and bored out of my mind. Each day was an internal battle. The future was a dreadful prospect; the anxious waiting for the next part of my body to break down was almost maddening. The present was something to be avoided, either with prescription pain pills that drained my energy and sapped my strength, but did little to actually numb the pain, or by smoking enough weed to disorient myself into forgetting how lonely I was. The latter always ended with me feeling disoriented and lonely. I quickly realized I had nothing to lose. How could I feel any worse than I felt right then? It was an epiphany. I had nothing to lose by giving faith a try. I decided to believe that God, or a benevolent spirit, or the communal soul, or whatever you want to call it, would guide me to health. I'd give it a two-month trial run. I'm not sure why I picked two months, it just seemed like a reasonable length of time to dedicate to such an endeavor back then. I told myself that for two months I would muster a die hard, unshakeable conviction that I would be healthy. For two months I would move past belief and know that I would be healthy and if after two months nothing had changed, fuck it, I could easily go back to being miserable, no problem.

I started right then. I said, "I am healthy, I am going to be healthy. I have faith in God, I am loved by God. I am healthy, I am going to be healthy" over and over again. I repeated those words out loud and in my head. I wrote them down. I filled every spare moment, of which I had no end, with those words. At the time I had a dualistic/Judeo-Christian view and these words reflect a belief that I was talking to something outside myself. This view was probably created by the unspoken influences of our society and the fact that I hadn't read much on the subject and what little thought I had dedicated didn't reach past the constraints of a Being "out there". Nevertheless I did everything in my power to know that my redundant mantra was true, that health was an inevitability for me. It wasn't easy. At first I felt like a liar, but I disregarded this. For the two-month experiment to be legitimate I had to have absolute, visceral, all encompassing faith. Otherwise I could just doubt that I hadn't committed myself enough. A funny thing happened within several days. I came to understand that when you let your guard down you can stand on it. Nothing changed physically, I still hurt all over, but I was happier than I had been in years. The pain would come but somehow it wouldn't devastate me the way it used to. I was able to rise above the pain easier than I ever had because I began to see the pain, and all things, through a lens of impermanence, and therefore was able to focus in on the present moment. I told myself I would be resilient and that nothing would stop me. With the burden of the future stripped away I could focus all my efforts on enjoying the present to whatever capacity of my abilities. I remember watching a boring baseball game and being engrossed by it. No longer did I worry how I would find happiness in the future if I barely had the strength to watch a game on TV. I would be healthy in the future so why not enjoy the game now.

I started praying to a spirit beyond myself. I had one-way dialogues where I thanked God for the beauty around me or the happiness inside me. The more I talked to the spirit the more I saw the spirit. This was the first gift the two-month experiment gave me because I started to see the celestial in everything around me. I'd long believed in the concept that everything was threaded into a vast, Holy fabric, that it was all held together by a benevolent force, but the more I talked to God and focused my attention on IT, the more I saw IT in everything. In trees. In the smiling face of a cashier. In the moon shooting through a crack of a curtain. Looking back I'm not really sure whom I was talking to. Was I talking to an omnipotent being completely outside of myself? Was I talking to a subtle causal consciousness deep within myself? I'm not sure it matters. The only two things that matter are that I was talking to something that transcended the limitations of my personal ego and that these conversations made me believe that some spiritual power cared for me and could aid my recovery if I gave It a chance by having faith.

Ken Wilber defines faith as something that "soldiers on when belief becomes unbelievable, for faith hears the faint but direct calling of a higher reality—of Spirit, of God, of Goddess, of Oneness—a higher reality that being beyond the mind is beyond belief." I like this interpretation, and I think that this is faith in the purest sense. Wilber is talking strictly in terms of enlightenment and liberation from the suffering caused by our mistaken identification with a dualistic reality. According to Wilber and many other mystics, beneath the surface of reality lies one underlying consciousness, an all-seeing witness, who is our true self. Experiential identification with that consciousness is enlightenment and faith is what draws us to discover this. Perhaps I stumbled into something less pure because my spirituality was tied together with my physical well being, but it was an excellent starting block for me and my eyes began to open.

The fear of being in pain had paralyzed me more and more in the past years. Early in the two-month experiment I started to shed this fear and gain confidence that I could overcome the pain and enjoy life despite of it. One night I decided to walk to the movies, which I hadn't done in months. It was about a twenty-minute walk, which was hard for me at the time, but I set off anyway. On the return walk it started to rain. I slowly marched through the cold, fall night and the drizzle soon turned into a downpour, drenching me as I plodded along. I was cold and wet. My legs ached and desperately begged me to stop walking. My back throbbed, my neck hurt, the cold rain whipped down. And I was elated. I was fucking elated. That's when I knew the experiment had worked. The end result didn't matter. It didn't matter whether I was ever healthy again or not. The act of having faith had connected me to a source of spirituality that I'd never known up until that point. I was alone and shivering, basically clawing my way up this hill in my neighborhood and my face was stuck in a grin. I couldn't stop smiling if I tried. I saw God's face everywhere; in the dripping trees whose droplets sparkled in the streetlights. In the swirling puddles that rushed by the drains. In the wonderful, pattering sound of the rain against the pavement and the patient, persistent drip of the tiny droplets that ran off the tip of my nose. The cracks of the road that spidered out into all sorts of captivating patterns. All of it was God. All of it was part of this majestic force that was so much greater than me, but included me as well. I'd understood the concept in the past, but now I felt it, I saw everything around me as a giant mosaic of the Divine. I was part of it too. Whatever flowed through these things around me and made them Holy, rushed through me too. My feet sloshed around in my frigid shoes, my hair was plastered to my face. I should have been miserable, and this thought made me erupt in laughter and I had to stop and compose myself as rain pelted down on me, washing away every impurity that could enter my mind. That feeling lasted for months, and for a while I thought that the rest of my life would be engulfed by such an overwhelming bliss. But it faded away some months later, and came back, and left again. It's something that I've always searched for ever since, even more than health. That form of elation that I felt walking home in the rain has turned into a barometer of whether I'm truly happy; because I was truly happy that night. I always kept the exhilaration I felt walking home from the movies in my pocket. It became the standard for how I wanted to carry myself and was the greatest gift of the two-month experiment.

Winter break was upon us. Lobo had been hounding me for weeks to come see him in Austin so we could spend Christmas in Mexico. And so on the 19th of December I packed the Honda once again and cut a southern route instead of my usual western one. I left DC right as the kids were being picked up from my school at three o'clock. We were all of us giddy with the prospect of two weeks off. I drove nine hours that day, stopping somewhere in Tennessee around midnight, then picked up again at dawn and rolled into Austin the following midnight. I didn't stop except to empty my bladder or refill the fuel tank, stacking a pile of sandwiches and drinks on the passenger seat to nourish me as I made my way deep into the south, past Nashville, Memphis, Little Rock, Dallas, and finally into Austin.

I was exhausted by the time I got to Lobo and Cassandra's bare apartment. I laid a camping pad down on their living floor and fell asleep instantly. The next morning Cassandra was cooking as Lobo played with his son. Cassandra is a beautiful, fair skinned Mexican woman, with long, thick, black hair, a round face, and dark eyes that peer quietly at all the movements around her. She is Lobo's wife, and also happens to be his first cousin. It sounds stranger than it is. When you're around them you see that they have real love for each other and that their union works on a deep, passionate level, and you forget everything else. Cassandra's father is Lobo's uncle, but after her parents separated her mother took her away from her father's side of the family, and subsequently Lobo rarely saw his striking cousin until they were teenagers. Their romance bloomed in their mid twenties when he moved back to Austin. Lobo having a child with his first cousin was merely the latest chapter in the utterly bizarre story that was his life. Now he had entered the select group of Edgar Allan Poe, Charles Darwin, and Albert Einstein, all of whom married their cousins.

We had big plans to drive to La Madrid, village of Lobo's ancestors, and spend the next week in Mexico, none of which came to fruition. Lobo's mother, Alejandra, and younger brother, Bruno, were staying with Lobo's uncle, (Cassandra's father), at the border town of Quemado. We were considering stopping by on the way to Mexico, but the visit was the topic of great debate in the morning because Cassandra was somewhat estranged from her father, and her father somewhat hated Lobo. "He blames me for the whole incest-baby thing," Lobo told me as we packed the car. "The last time I saw him was at a family reunion in La Madrid about two months ago. Man, shit got fucked up, but it was all my fault. You see I haven't had a one on one with that fellow since Cassandra got pregnant. You know I miss him, he was always my favorite uncle, but he won't talk to me. I knew the only way to get him to talk to me was to fuck with him. You know he left Cassandra when she was four, that's why I never really met her until we were sixteen or something. Anyways, I started blaming the whole thing on him, you see. It was all his fault. If he hadn't left his family Cassandra and me would have grown up together and we wouldn't have a baby now. I pounded him with insults, 'you left your children, you traded your children for a car and then left in it,' I said to him and more. Then he charged me and took a swing at me, but I knew he was coming because that's what I was aiming for, and I dodged him, asking him to be faster, 'Mas rapido.' I taunted him, but I never hit him. His girlfriend pulled us apart and he left. Man, I felt real bad about it then. Next day he showed up at my mother's house and in his own way wanted to bury the hatchet. He brought breakfast and wanted to know if he was still welcome in the house. I ran up and gave him a hug and apologized. He said fine, but was still all distant from me. Every now and then he'd glance at me and say, 'Go fuck your mother,' which is his sister, but he's said that a million times to a million people, so I guess it was habit. He told me that I move like a grasshopper, but next time he'll catch me with his 45. 'Pow,'." Lobo formed a gun with his fingers as he finished his sentence.

Cassandra's father was the craziest of the De Los Reyes clan, a sort of patriarch of chaos, intensity, and fire. He had passed something wild to his nephew through both the science of genetics and the spark of inspiration. When Lobo spoke of him there was a reverence in his tone that I'd never heard him use for anyone before. "You just don't know what he's gonna do...ever. One minute everything is good and he's laughing and hunky dory, and the next minute he'll explode into an animal, ready to end you"

Lobo and I were both geared up for the thrill of running into this madman, but were conscious that in the end it was Cassandra's decision. A man like this wins no father-of-the-year awards and though I never got a clear picture of exactly what went down, I was able to deduce that he'd left Cassandra's mother for her best friend, had two more kids with the new woman, then left her too. Lobo tried to contain his excitement by speaking in hushed murmurs that tapered off anytime Cassandra breezed by. "What do you think babe?" he asked once the car was properly packed.

"I don't know," Cassandra answered, visibly conflicted over the prospect. "He's been calling me all the time, he wants, to like, talk to me now. I haven't answered most of his calls. It's weird. He's weird. I don't want to talk to him...on the phone."

"Yes, yes," Lobo nodded at every word.

In the end Cassandra opted to go see her father on our way to La Madrid, but only to stay for a quick lunch. Four hours south of Austin we found ourselves in the tiny, borderland town of Quemado. Against the gravel crust of a single lane highway that runs a mile from Mexico was a small, scraggly plot of dusty brush land. "I don't even know how he got this land," Lobo told me as we pulled up. "Probably some under the table deal with someone and now he just lives here. He's got plots like these all over Texas, I think." There were two gutted RV trailers and a small pen for animals that was empty. A motor home, in slightly better condition, stood between the trailers and acted as his house. Lobo's mother, Alejandra, was there by herself. Her legendary brother was off working with Lobo's younger brother, Bruno. "He has these mini ponies," Lobo elaborated, "like about eight of them and a livestock trailer and whenever he runs out of money he takes them to whatever flea market he's around and sets them up, charging five bucks for kids to ride around in a circle, ten bucks with a crappy Polaroid of the kid on the pony. He cleans up too. He can haul over 1,000 bucks in a good weekend. Around here everyone knows him as the man with the ponies. That's where him and Bruno are now."

The sun was out but the cold winter wind ran over the plains, cutting chills into us as it whistled through the short, barren trees. Alejandra and I built a fire. Cassandra found an old tattered American flag and unrolled it next to the fire as a tarp. I came upon an old window screen, which we set on blocks around the fire for a grill. We ate the chicken we cooked with our hands, grease running through our fingers, wiping our hands on whatever rags we could find in our cars or on the premises. There was no other way. The lord of the manor had no use for plates or silverware. "My uncle has no shame or conformity," Lobo boasted as he wiped his hands on his jeans.

I took a walk around the place and started to get a sense of the hardened ogre that lived there. Assorted piles of scrap metal and broken, abandoned tools lay in scattered mounds within the dusty, desert weeds. A shabby, torn Jacuzzi, half filled with water, acted as his fridge now that the cold winter months had arrived. The sole inhabitant was a half filled jug of milk listlessly floating amongst some leaves. Around the corner was a tiny shed. This shed, believe it or not, acted as his dentistry office. Somehow, someway this man had acquired some crude dentistry skill and performed dental work on those unfortunate enough to be unable to afford anyone else. He specialized in dentures mostly. The shed was as dirty as any place else on his land. A swivel lamp was attached to a tray on a mini fridge that held some dentist's tools, looking like something out of a horror movie. A set of broken dentures lay on the floor. "People say he's actually pretty good," Lobo offered with a shrug.

Several hours later, as dusk began and the first bold stars peered in the still, blue sky, the legend arrived. A prophetic cloud loomed at his back, looking just like fire in both shape and color, inflaming the western horizon. I was captivated by this cloud, and barely noticed the old red pickup, with a long metal livestock trailer in tow, maneuvering into the grounds. Lobo later told me, "When I turned around and saw that cloud I thought it was going to reach out and grab me like a hand. I saw it and my life was changed for a second, and then it was back to usual."

The "back to usual" was probably the thunderous voice of his uncle cracking across the plains. Lobo sprang into action and started leading ponies off the trailer along with his younger brother. The old man pointed at me and I made my way to the truck. "Rene De Los Reyes," he said with emphatic purpose, sticking out his grimy, calloused hand. Rene was a stocky man, with grey stubble, a salt and pepper mustache, and a dusty green trucker's cap fitted on his head. He walked as if he was cutting through something at all times. His black eyes glared even when he smiled. His thick shoulders hunched over into his beaten leather jacket. He made his way to Cassandra and scuffed his boot into the dusty gravel as he talked, somewhat awkwardly, with the daughter that he'd lost touch with. Cassandra wasn't making things easy for him. Her soft, dark eyes followed her son, or the ponies, or anything other than her father. Her face was stone like, as if she were talking to a stranger she was wary of. After some time she went off with her son. Rene moved to Alejandra and Lobo, invoking rounds of laughter at the end of his stories. From the little Spanish I understood I could tell that he was quite charismatic in his own, barbaric way, much like his nephew.

But Rene was cold to his nephew, and Lobo in turn became quiet, almost bashfully shy. I was used to seeing him addicted to the spotlight, but now he deferred to Tio Rene. At one point we were standing around the fire pit when Rene asked Lobo if he'd placed the feed bucket with the ponies and Lobo instinctively lied that he had. Rene leaned over and saw no bucket feed and shot his nephew murderous daggers from his black marble eyes as a snarl of curses erupted from his mouth. Lobo quickly ran to remedy the situation. At this point Cassandra abruptly announced that it was time for us to continue south into Mexico and we packed up to leave. Alejandra and Bruno were heading north to San Antonio. Rene stood like a statue as the procession of his family lined up to hug him goodbye. He looked coldly into the distance, his hands buried deep within his pockets, as each person hugged him then moved on, making no sign that he'd even noticed their presence. Cassandra came last and he remained frozen until she confronted him, "come on Papa," in a voice that implored and reprimanded simultaneously. He thawed and briefly wrapped an arm around her.

We left for Mexico in the night, rolling effortlessly through the Eagle Pass border crossing, cutting past all the border town traffic and neon billboard signs, and running deep into the dark, bleak, deserted night. 90 minutes down the road we came upon a checkpoint. I had to get my passport stamped and Lobo had to register the car with the Mexican government. I paid my fee and strolled back to the car. Lobo trudged back with a despondent scowl on his face and broke the bad news to us. "He says he won't let us in without the registration. It's the same guy from the last two times and he remembers us."

"Shit," Cassandra said. They began the futile search for the papers they both knew had been lost months ago. The last two times they'd taken their car into Mexico they had to sweet talk this very agent into letting them pass without the correct documents and this time he wasn't budging. There was nothing left to do but get back in the car and head back. "Fuck," Lobo bellowed behind the wheel. "That piece of shit, worthless motherfucker, I wanna run that cocksucker down right now God damn it..." and on like this as we wearily drove back toward Eagle Pass, deflated by bureaucracy a mere forty miles from the cozy comforts of La Madrid—six hours south of home at ten o' clock in the evening with no place to go but north.

At four in the morning he pulled up an hour short of Austin at his mother's house in San Antonio. The next day was Christmas Eve. Lobo and I went to Austin to fetch my car, bringing the Honda back to San Antonio to fully prepare for another run into Mexico in two days. We had to wait until the 26th for the DMV to open so Cassandra and Lobo could procure the correct papers for the authorities across the border.

We were waiting for the DMV express to open on the morning of the 26th. Within five minutes we were south bound with all the correct papers. Lobo had lobbied for a return visit to Quemado, and after some persuasion Cassandra had relented. The plan was simple enough, though somewhat of a grind for me. We would drive back to Quemado and have lunch with Rene. I would follow them in the Honda. A brief lunch was all that Cassandra seemed comfortable with and Lobo was sensitive not to push for more. From there we'd go to La Madrid where I would stay for exactly one night before racing back to DC by New Year's Eve for my friend's show that I didn't want to miss.

Upon arrival in Quemado Rene dragged Cassandra to the store, returning with a giant, greasy plastic sack of seasoned ribs. He plopped the sack onto a lawn table, threw a smaller bag with tortillas next to it, then stuck his dirty hand into the meat, tearing off a chunk, slapping it into a tortilla and stuffing the whole thing into his mouth. I was starving and reached my hand into the sack too. But I tried to tenderly tear a piece without getting my fingers on everyone else's meat. "Con tu manos, hijo," Rene bellowed at me—with your hands, son. I quickly and eagerly took my queue, digging my fingers in and ripping off a hearty chunk. We ate lunch in this grand way as they talked in Spanish and laughed, Rene and Lobo uproariously, Cassandra softly. Rene was holding court, telling one story after another, and even though I couldn't understand them I knew they were latent, filthy, macho, comic masterpieces. I could see these stories of his reach into Cassandra and produce a reluctant chuckle when they were especially funny. When Lobo would laugh a little too hard Rene would snarl at him, and then continue.

The topic of my drive to Mexico with Lobo and Cassandra came up. I was planning to drive three hours south only to leave the next morning and begin the long ride north to DC. Rene was outraged by the stupidity of it all. "He says you're an idiot for going down with us," Lobo informed me, translating his uncle's rants. "He says if there was a woman waiting for you it would be another thing, then you should drive five hours to stay fifteen minutes. But with no woman, fuck it." Then Lobo paused for a second as if trying to process the old man's last sentence. "He wants you to stay here with him tonight and leave for DC in the morning," he told me almost stunned. "You should do it, it's too much driving for you."

The idea of staying out there with someone that even Lobo considered to be a lunatic was somewhat intimidating, but I also couldn't deny that it made sense. "That's cool," I blurted out before I could stop myself, "I'll crash here." When Lobo told his Uncle, Rene smiled broadly and through a series of hand gestures indicated that we were going to have a fine night. Then, as if to solidify the point, he walked over to welcome me, but unable to use any language he just came out and hugged me. It was the manliest, back-thumping-est hug in history.

"Are you sure?" Cassandra asked me, her face a mixture of concern and surprise.

"It'll be fine," I responded. Rene suggested that they all sleep on his land tonight but Cassandra shook her head no. He insisted once more as Lobo's eyes perked, but she flatly and coldly refused. She barely said goodbye, walking to the car and waiting in the passenger seat as Lobo said his goodbyes to me and Rene. And with that Lobo, Cassandra, and Junior got into their car and left. Rene gave me a quick tour of his RV, showed me where I would sleep and promptly laid down to take a nap.

And that was the extent of my stay alone with Tio Rene. About twenty minutes later I heard the churn of tires on gravel and stepped out of the RV to see Lobo and Cassandra pull up. "We're staying here tonight too," Lobo triumphantly announced. I could tell that he had spurred their return, that he didn't want to miss a chance to smooth things over with his uncle now that the old man was feeling so sociable. Our chatter awoke Rene and he stumbled out, rubbing his thick head then pulling his cap low over his brow. When they told him they were staying for the night he smiled for a second before vanishing to the shed and returning with a rifle, barking orders for us to get into the truck. Cassandra and junior sat up in the cabin with Rene, and Lobo and I eased into the bed as the truck grumbled, then roared off.

"I know it sounds crazy, but I could be holding my future here," Lobo solemnly stated, looking at the rifle in his hands as we sped down the narrow highway. His face had an anxious twist to it, as if he now regretted the decision to come back. We turned on a dirt road and left billowing trails of dust clouds behind us. "I know it's 99 out of 100 going to be fine, but I wouldn't put it past him to drive me out here and shoot me." He was somber as he spoke, staring intently at the gun like he was trying to make peace with it. I didn't know who was crazier, Lobo for indulging such paranoid thoughts or the uncle for having such a fierce reputation that his nephew wasn't completely at ease with his life around him. Probably both were equally nuts. He drove us deep into a barren, dusty land. Desert plains stretched in all directions. He popped out from behind the wheel and grabbed some bottles that were scattered about the bed of the truck, then jogged off some twenty yards away and set up a mini firing range. When he came back he took the first couple of shots before handing the rifle to Lobo, while leading Cassandra away to talk. I got the sense he was trying not to be such an ogre with her. His look was not as cast away, and his hands weren't so fiercely dug into his pockets. He seemed to ponder his words a little longer as the two of them stared out into the vast horizon. Maybe he was talking about the weather, or the truck, or the gun. Maybe his words weren't amounting to anything significant, but he seemed to be allowing the meager trivialities that found their way out of his mouth into the air with the hope that they'd build into something more.

He yelled at me and Lobo to load the truck with the dead logs that lay in piles around the dried up shrubs. Lobo hauled armfuls of wood into the truck with a near panicked vigor. The sooner we got out of the barren no man's land the better. When the bed was full I hopped in. Rene grabbed the rifle from his nephew, took one more shot at a bottle, then snarled a smile as he returned the gun and slid behind the wheel. We cut on back through the dust toward his land and Lobo held the gun a little more confidently as we raced. I could vaguely see the makings of a magical night brewing ahead of us. I could sense what everyone wanted out of the evening and almost see all the different outcomes each of us subconsciously hoped for converging right around the corner. I wanted a timeless and soulful instant. Junior wanted to be with his parents. We were the easy ones to please. Lobo, Rene and Cassandra were tangled in something deeper and more complex, a sort of merry-go-round of reconciliation. But they too were on this track to converge at this one point, on this one night. And all of us, with our petty needs and grievances were blindly barreling toward this point around the bend, where for one night things would just work out and we could all rest peacefully until we diverged and scattered, dismantling what we knew couldn't stand the weight of its own construction for long.

We stopped by the store and got some chicken, potatoes and vegetables. By the time we got back to the trailers and the ponies, darkness blanketed the land and a cold, winter chill cut across the plain in murmurous howls. Cooking supplies were low to say the least. I had two camping pots and a mini butane burner in my trunk and Rene rummaged around his shed and produced one beaten, dented pot and a propane burner from the ruble. With these humble tools Cassandra went about to cook a delicious chicken soup while Lobo and I built a fire big enough to stave off the quickly dropping temperature. We only had two small pots to serve as bowls so we ate in shifts. Cassandra and Junior ate first as I sat by the fire and played my guitar. Lobo and Rene sat across from me, talking magnanimously to each other. Their hoarse laughter, grunts, and Spanish banter accompanied my guitar almost like a song. The campfire crackled as the sweet smell of burning wood seeped into our clothes. All these celestial sounds flurried and fluttered up into the cold, black night—the symphony of the fire and the guitar, the cold night and the hot soup, the stars and the vague reconciliation that was simultaneously being plodded through and mapped out between both Lobo and Rene, and Rene and Cassandra, all mixed together harmoniously into something perfect that we were all aimlessly stumbling upon.

Cassandra went to bed with Junior. Rene ran ahead of them to the motor home and set up the rear bedroom as nicely as he could. He plugged in a space heater and gave them a mound of blankets. He then promptly converted one of the gutted trailers, which had looked like an uninhabitable heap of metal, into a cozy little spot for himself by boarding up the openings and laying down a set of blankets on the bare floor. There was room for Lobo in the motor home but he announced that he was sleeping by the fire. I had already laid the back seats down in the Honda, so everyone's quarters were set for the night. Soon after Cassandra retired the old man hit the sack. Lobo and I stayed up talking.

The temperature dropped to the mid twenties and we threw one log into the fire after the other. Lobo shared his belief that had fate not brought Cassandra into his life he was sure that he and Rene would have toured both Mexico and the U.S. with those ponies, setting up shop in every small town along the way and cleaning up in the process. He said this in a mournful tone, but in the end he knew he was a family man more than a rambler, just like Rene was a rambler more than a family man. I think each man enviously looked at what the other had despite knowing they were better suited for the individual roles they had fallen into. I strummed a simple folk song, one of the first I had written, and Lobo hummed an inspired, wordless tune. At times his voice rose into moans and he sounded like some form of majestic animal. My hands grew tired and I put the guitar down. He muttered something I could barely hear. It sounded like "thank you," as he stared at the embers. I don't know who or what he was talking to. The night got colder and colder as the fire labored away. "Do you think they're all jealous of us?" Lobo asked as he stared vacantly into the fire.

"Who?"

"All of them, the whole crew from Umass."

"I don't know," I answered. "Probably not, but they should be." This seemed to satisfy Lobo and he resumed his vacant staring. The night had picked up steam from some hidden location and had rushed by with a fumbling, poetic quality. We were all characters in the production, stumbling down our own paths and unwittingly conspiring to string together something beautiful and timeless, like a piece of art that resounds inside you long after you've first seen it. I didn't think our friends were sensitive to those kinds of emotions anymore, and subsequently the beauty of it all would have been missed to them.

Lobo took the flag that Cassandra had used as a tarp several days ago and folded it into his own stars and stripes pillow. He marked his resting place for the night by the fire, inching closer and closer to the embers while curling up into a sad, blanket-less ball. It was a brutally cold night, and when we woke up we found holes in the back of his shirt where the coals had burned through as he kept inching toward the fire pit. I had a sleeping bag in the car and slept with every article of clothing I could find on, as my legs stretched into the trunk and my head rested by the front seats.

In the frozen dawn I found a package of pancake mix buried in the Honda. The milk was a solid block of ice and we had to let it thaw before mixing a batch of cakes, then frying them on a sheet of metal over the fire. Junior and I hopped the fence and picked pecans from the neighbor's farm, cracking them open with our teeth while we waited. All five of us sat around the fire and ate the dry pancakes in the frosty, morning glow. Rene and Cassandra saddled Junior onto a pony and led him on a ride around the frost-covered plot. The three of them posed for pictures as Lobo handled the camera. Cassandra smiled as her father wrapped his arm around both of them. Soon it was go time. Rene protested, but there was no fighting it. We all knew this was a one-night affair. A line formed to bid farewell to the old man. He kissed his grandson and his daughter. Hugged his nephew and shook my hand. Lobo, Cassandra and Junior headed south while I cut a northern route to DC. Rene stoically stood in the driveway smiling, while still finding a way to scowl beneath the surface, perpetually disgusted by something he could never identify.

I'd like to say that the night had changed everything between Rene and his daughter, as well as Rene and his nephew, but things are never that simple. In the years to come Rene remained as unreliable and unpredictable as ever. He blew chances to build goodwill with Cassandra by skipping his second grandson's birthday and the unofficial wedding that Cassandra and Lobo held for each other a little more than a year later. He would still show up unannounced at their house in Austin from time to time, sometimes laughing with Lobo affably, only to bark like an angry dog at him immediately thereafter. One such trip he arrived from some lonely flea market when Lobo had taken his family out camping for the weekend, and all that was left of him when they returned was a blue heeler puppy tied to a post in the backyard and a box in the cellar that read "live grenades" on it.

Lab Results
October 12, 2000

My body had been all sorts of banged up for almost three years. Starting with a perplexing headache at the end of 1997, things had deteriorated to the point where I could barely stand in the fall of 2000. One body part failed after another. Pain moved down my body like an inverted flood, leaking down from my neck, to my back and hands, and finally to my legs. During that time I had marched down a procession of doctors, all of who had either dismissed my symptoms as psychosomatic or offered little more than painkillers and shrugs. No one could tell me what was wrong and what to do about it.

About a month ago I had read a book that convinced me to give faith a try. For some reason I took an almost clinical perspective and decided to treat an exercise in faith like an experiment. I gave the whole thing two months. For two months I would force myself to believe that I would be healthy. I would force myself to go past belief and know that I would find a way to shed all the pain that constricted my movements throughout the day. For two months I would know that I was destined to enjoy the liberties of a fully functional body. There were several pay offs early into the experiment that had little to do with my actual physical condition, but more to do with my outlook on life and health. One night, after a long drought, happiness bloomed in an arduous walk in the rain.

A month after starting my experiment I waited in a doctor's office deeming my trail run in faith a success for the simple reason that I was happy. I hadn't said that in years. And then something remarkable happened. After nearly three years of doctor's visits, three years of glib dismissals of my symptoms, three years of confounded looks and the same tired suggestions—never once producing a diagnosis as to what was wrong with my body, I got one. I remember waiting in the doctor's room, staring at posters of lung disease, saying my little mantra over and over again, (*I am going to be healthy, I am...*). The doctor said she wanted to do a Lyme disease test. I'd actually had one done a year ago, a spinal tap up at the Mayo clinic, which had come back negative, but she said it was worth a second try. You see Lyme disease is a controversial thing, and what one doctor considers a negative test another considers positive. The test came back positive several days later.

I got a phone call from the doctor's office with the news. At first I was blown away, and even a little scared. Could it really be this easy? Three years I'd been searching for an answer as to what was wrong with me, as to why my body was falling apart and no one could give me any answers, and one month into my two-month experiment in faith I got the diagnosis that had been eluding me all along? A surreal jolt buzzed around my stomach as I processed what the doctor had told me.

The timing of the diagnosis may have been a coincidence, it may not have been. It may have been tied together with the experiment or it may have been a case of random parallelism. Personally I think our thoughts are capable of much more than we're aware of and if you can find the right rhythm, the right balance of determination and detachment, your thoughts can shape reality much the same way water wears away at a stone, patiently smoothing over the surface initially, then eventually impressing its path into the rock. The day I got the diagnosis the doctor told me I'd be starting an antibiotic regiment later that week. I thought I'd be playing basketball in a month, though it took almost three years. And once I got healthy enough to lift weights again I thought I was done with this particular challenge in life, though it reappeared in my life again several times. And though I'd often get deflated when I'd fall into a relapse of a disease that just refuses to let go of its grip on my system, in turn I refuse to let go of what the two month experiment taught me. Fourteen years down the line in this experiment on faith and positive thinking I'm not naive enough to think that things are as simple as "will it one day and reap the benefits the next," but I'm also not jaded to the point where I lose sight of the invisible play that our thoughts have on reality. Lab results keep coming in everyday, we've just got to read the correct interpretation.

Calculated Risk
July 5–July 23, 2007

Several weeks after losing the Honda in Oakland I arrived at Austin international airport around one in the morning. Costa and I had rented a car and made the best of it in the Bay area, driving a little loop around northern California that ended at San Francisco airport. Costa flew home to DC, and I jumped on a plane to Texas. After retrieving my bags I made several phone calls to Lobo, trying to keep my cool as each one went to voice mail. I wondered if I'd end up sleeping in the airport as Lobo's drunken dreams of something he was supposed to do haunted him throughout the night. I reached him on my fourth try and saw the Toyota Matrix he'd recently purchased pull up soon after. Enter Lobo into my summer, the mad Mexican drunk on life and everything else. He plodded out to meet me with his signature, crooked grin and helped me with my bags. A stranger sat in the front seat so I stepped in the back.

I settled into the back seat and observed Lobo and this stranger. His name was Kinglin. He was a skinny white guy with short brown hair and a ragged yellow t-shirt. They were both teachers in the same school, both off for the summer, and both sipping on Coronas as we sped down the interstate. "Kinglin's goin' to Mexico with us," Lobo said. The more the merrier was always his first instinct.

"Yeah, after that I'm moving to Chicago," Kinglin vaulted in. "I'm actually homeless right now," he continued in a slurred, braggart's voice. "My roommate shipped to Iraq and I got no place to stay until I move in with my mother in Chicago. All my shit is split up between Lobo's place, my buddy's down in San Antonio and my car." Apparently he'd been sleeping in anyone of these places for the past weeks.

Lobo and Cassandra's apartment was a dwelling void of any furniture aside from a table with four chairs neatly resting in one corner next to the kitchen and a bed in the bedroom. Kinglin trudged through the piles of his belongings that cluttered the entrance, balled up a blanket into a pillow and fell asleep on his back, like a stiff board, motionless and rigidly straight. He was becoming an inconvenience to his hosts, though he had no idea at the time, and would only figure it out after it was too late.

I grabbed Lobo's guitar. I hadn't held one since mine was stolen and it felt wonderful in my hands. "Check this out Lobo, it's one I made up before I left DC." My fingers reacquainted themselves with a lost love. Lobo nodded his head like an ancient professor and spoke in low, deep tones, "That's nice Vittas, that's real nice." I knew I should have felt tired, but now some hidden reserve of energy kicked in and sleep was impossible. The two of us spoke in the hushed, violent whispers we always used when trying not to wake up Junior, occasionally frothing into an outburst of laughter. We talked mostly of what we would do in Austin, and then in Mexico. Lobo was aching to take me back to La Madrid, ranting in his excited, meandering way about the last month he and the boy spent down there while Cassandra stayed in Austin, working and taking night classes. Cassandra always was a sweetheart and I'd built a close friendship with her when we all spent the previous summer traveling through California as a family. Lobo rambled on. "Oh Nick, I can't wait 'til we get down there, I put up a pull-up bar on the side porch of my Mom's place. I've been getting' all buff. I hired this guy and together we poured concrete into half of the pool, like a ledge, because it was too deep for my son to go into before. Now I just gotta smooth that part out, clean the rest of it and that baby will be open for the summer." Cassandra woke up and the party moved into the bedroom. We bantered as quietly as possible over the sleeping child. Lobo slapped and poked me. Cassandra sat cross-legged on her bed, dark eyes darting back and forth between us, following the volleys of stories like a tennis match.

The next morning all the excitement of the night was gone. Cassandra and Lobo continued an ongoing fight. Well really Lobo continued it. You could never say that he feared confrontation. He was incensed that he came back from his month in Mexico to a messy apartment. "You had a whole month," he lit into her nastily, "and look, I guess this is how you want to live. I guess you enjoy living in filth. I guess you enjoy having your son wallow in filth." The onslaught of sarcastic, mean spirited comments was endless and hard to watch.

"I was depressed," she said. "You can't leave me alone and take Baby again." Her pleas were only returned with insults.

"You're a filth pig, a god damned, Indian, filth pig." When he pushed her enough Cassandra fought back, voicing her objections in Spanish. Even though I couldn't understand everything she said the basics of her message were *clean the house yourself, asshole.* Lobo could barely contain his frustration, pleading to the ceiling, "I can't argue with her, it's like arguing with a dumb animal, an animal that is dumb and lives in the woods."

That's the thing with Lobo, he makes no apologies for who he is and what he wants. He can callously rip into his wife, his brother, even his mother without a second thought. Maybe he's always betting that the natural inclination humans have to let go of grievances will play itself out, and the offended party will forgive him sooner or later. Or maybe he just doesn't give a damn. Or maybe he just has an innate understanding that sensitivities don't hold any real weight in the grand scheme of things and he's done away with them altogether. His ability to bluntly and forcibly move those around him is a trait I've been envious of at times. I just don't have it in me. When he turns his rancor on someone else it's uncomfortable, when it's turned on you it's downright awful. I felt for Cassandra in that moment, but I said nothing.

I quietly hung my head in the corner as they quarreled, wondering why I had dragged myself down here again. Wasn't the madness of driving across the west with him last summer enough for me? Why had I linked up with this lunatic once again? And to make things worse, this summer we were slated to drive through Mexico, his land, where he would inevitably fall into the position of control. I didn't even know what that implied, I just knew a certain degree of instability automatically came attached with any ship that Lobo was the captain of. The swell of belonging that had engulfed me the night before vanished as I heard Lobo bellow and rant.

The tension between Cassandra and Lobo blew over by the next day. As angry as he got with his wife, he really loved her and couldn't stay angry for long. And as savagely as he acted toward her, Cassandra adored him, and usually forgave him sooner or later. Lobo and I spent the rest of the week running around Austin, catching cheap blues shows off the 6th street strip. One of the nights Lobo and I were out listening to music we got a frantic phone call from Cassandra. Apparently a drunken Kinglin, slurring his words and reeking of booze, thumped on the apartment door like a madman at one in the morning. He trudged around in his muddy boots, thinking perhaps that he was in a college shit house rather than a family apartment with a three year old sleeping in the next room. Cassandra was a bit rattled, and very angry, when she called us, which was right after she threw him out. Lobo called Kinglin and I saw the fire of confrontation ignite in him as he feverishly ripped into Kinglin, screaming at him in the most demeaning way imaginable. "What the fuck is wrong with you? How the fuck am I goin' to take you to Mexico if you don't know how to act for Christ's sake? Are you a fuckin' retard or just an idiot?"

By the next day Cassandra had flatly proclaimed that she wouldn't go anywhere with Kinglin, and so he was thrown out of the trip to Mexico. Lobo now had leeway to begin the long, drawn out process of berating Kinglin until he didn't want to come. He relished this with evil glee and called Kinglin immediately. "Kinglin you're an idiot, it's okay. I shouldn't let you come to Mexico, but I will...if you don't drink even one beer the whole trip and are in bed by 10:30 no matter what, then you can come." When Kinglin threw up objections to these ridiculous stipulations Lobo mockingly chastised him like a child. "Kinglin, these are the consequences when you barge into my house and terrify my wife. No booze. Bed by 10:30, take it or leave it. And you probably shouldn't speak unless spoken to. I mean God knows what may fly out of that idiot mouth of yours. I'm a family man, you could get me killed with your stupidity. We're not going to a merry-go-round; we're going to Mexico. Am I wrong?" By the end, when Kinglin came to get the rest of his stuff, I felt sorry for him. His blue eyes trembled like they were about to shatter and it was all a joke to Lobo; it was always a joke to Lobo. He kept laying it on thick, asking Kinglin on his way out, "well, that's cool you don't want to go and all, but you got any weed you can give me?" He was actually serious, and would have snatched a bag of weed out of Kinglin's hand had he offered it.

"What? No. No." Kinglin was flabbergasted. "You're throwing me out and asking me for weed? No. No." He slammed the door and left as Lobo laughed maniacally, like a villain.

Lobo was more volatile this summer than the last. A jaded brutality seemed to fester in him, bursting out at odd times. He had enjoyed dragging Kinglin over the coals. And even though the confrontation with Cassandra lacked the celebratory, sportsman like air that his conflict with Kinglin took, some valve within him was releasing stress during his argument with her too. I watched him from an uneasy distance. I couldn't really tell when the next eruption was coming. We were slated to leave for Mexico in a couple of days.

Directly after Kinglin's departure, Dan, our buddy from Umass, called and asked if he could jump on board the trip through Mexico. Lobo's attitude is always the more the merrier, and Dan showed up with his girlfriend Linda at the Greyhound bus station from Boston, 52 grueling hours later. Their arrival made our trip to Mexico slightly more complicated now that there was only one car between me, Lobo, Cassandra, Junior, Linda, and Dan. There was only one car, Lobo and Cassandra's compact Toyota Matrix, because my Honda had been stolen in Oakland, Kinglin's car was no longer available, and "Miracle Blue" didn't have the tires for a long trip this summer. Nonetheless we sped down highway 57 stuffed in the compact car the next day and crossed the border at Eagle Pass. Cassandra's father was probably rounding up his mini ponies nearby, though I wouldn't meet him until the winter.

We spent the next week in La Madrid, the tiny village of Lobo and Cassandra's roots, in relative peace. There was a night when we went to the wrestling matches in the nearest town of Monclova, and he became belligerently drunk. The savage atmosphere of the arena, along with the cheap beer, sowed the seeds for an ugly episode to ensue afterwards where he got into it with some of Cassandra's cousins from her mother's side. After a senseless argument the night ended with Lobo slouched in a chair by the house, legs sloppily stretched out, a bottle of tequila in one hand, a bottle of beer in the other, in some kind of drunkard's peaceful protest. Still, for the most part it was smooth and mellow in La Madrid, which was great, but I wanted more.

Earlier in the spring, when Lobo and I would discuss our summer plans over the phone, there had been talk of a mad dash across Mexico when I made it down to him, but these grand ideas were slipping away. I tried to push the subject when I could. Lobo had a strange resistance to it and I couldn't figure out why. But I also couldn't let it go. His eyes shot back at me a couple of times, and I'd pull back, wary of rattling the bear's cage too hard. One week turned into two, and it seemed we would stay planted in the village because of lack of space in the car, lack of funds, lack of time, and lack of motivation from anyone else but me.

Still, the idea of navigating through the treasure chest of Mexico was too tantalizing an idea to let go of. I brought the idea up again, cornering Lobo on a walk to the store as dusk bathed the village. He offered several tense excuses for not embarking, but I shot everyone down until it was agreed that Dan, Linda, Lobo, and I would depart on the 23rd of July for a tour of the country. Cassandra hadn't expressed interest in going, and I told Lobo that I'd pay his way until the first of the month, when his paycheck would be direct deposited. But, there was an undercurrent of tension surrounding the plan. At first I thought Lobo was projecting Cassandra's objections to this arrangement, but as the date of departure approached I could tell something didn't sit right with Lobo. None of us thwarted the development of our plans, and slowly the day of departure arrived under a cloak of unresolved, unidentified tension.

On the morning of the 23rd Dan, Linda, and I packed our bags and waited through three mock departures as Lobo agonized in the hammock, in the bedroom, in the kitchen, anywhere but toward the car. It took an hour and a half to get him into the driver's seat. He quietly fumed as he made his way. He was visibly angry and I felt sick because no one is more vindictive when they're angry than Lobo, and there was an undercurrent of discontent pointed straight at me, the one who was taking him away from his family. Lobo is an open faucet, when he's feeling good he can fill the world with smiles, and when he's pissed off he can spew a litany of hurtful, malicious comments aimed at maiming the people around him as if it were a sport. Often these scalding remarks are so over the top and ridiculous that they're almost funny, except for how deeply he intends them to strike.

His dark eyes glowered and his wide nose flared and when he's like this a toxic field forms around him and no one wants to go near him. I'd seen this nasty side of him many times, a couple in the last week. This was the animal I had boiling next to me as we prepared to take our tour through the guts of Mexico. He was so ugly. Perhaps I had been blind and head strong in my desire to roam Mexico rather than stay planted in La Madrid, but it was too late now.

Cassandra and Junior waved to us from the porch as we rolled down the gravel road. Their round faces, Junior's dark like his daddy's, Cassandra's slightly lighter, smiled sadly in the doorway. The car was still with an uncomfortable silence and lacked any sign of the expected excitement at the beginning of a trip. Lobo scowled behind the wheel with a sarcastic smile smeared across his face; it was awful. A wounded, "whoo-hoo," slipped out of Dan, sliding out in a vain attempt to spark the emotion that was clearly lacking in the car. I wondered what the fuck train wreck I had put myself on and lamented that there was no way out now that the wheels were moving. Lobo could easily turn the next week into a vindictive, excruciating affair that I'd have to endure. And worst of all, the seething, grim faced statue brooding behind the wheel would be a pleasantry compared to the belligerent beast I'd have to deal with after a couple of beers made their way down his gullet. We rounded one corner and pulled to a stop.

"Let's give it one more try," Lobo muttered, spinning the car back toward the house. At this point I was grateful that the runaway train had been derailed, at least for the moment. He asked Cassandra if she wanted to come. Her cute brow furrowed and she said no. He asked her again. She looked out to the mountains and said maybe. He asked her one more time and she agreed to come and we all piled out of the car. We had some logistical problems to ponder, like who would be riding in the hatch back trunk or whether it was practical to ride through Mexico with bags attached to the roof rack, but at least Lobo's scowl was gone. Nothing good can happen when that look is prodding him along.

We all sat and looked at the compact Toyota we had as a vehicle for this proposed trip like it was a puzzle we needed to figure out. Cassandra blurted out that we all could fit, if each person only brought one change of clothes and a bathing suit. "We'll leave right now, Nick," Cassandra told me, her black eyes beaming from her saucer face. "We're not taking the roof rack because it's gonna get stolen, so everyone is only allowed to bring the clothes they're wearing and a bathing suit."

"I'm not even going to wear any clothes," Lobo boasted. In a complete reversal, the cup of his soul was now swelling with laughter, splashing a roaring glee about him with the rhythm and force of the Colorado rapids.

"No, we all have to wear red shirts," Dan added in chipper sarcasm, mocking the military tone of these slightly panicked, sensational rules. His large frame bounded with agile precision to the car to unload the trunk. Cassandra had been the general behind this sudden movement. Ten minutes later I was in a car that brimmed with good spirits. A half-filled backpack containing three pairs of underwear, a spare shirt, my journal, and all my pills lay at my feet. Cassandra's enthusiasm had spearheaded the journey, steamrolling far ahead, clearing the path of any negativity, so we could glide on down. We ate a late lunch at Monclova, laughing at the fact that through the whole process it took us six hours to travel 60 miles.

We fled Monclova and into new territory that was virgin to my eyes. Dan, Lobo, and Junior snored lightly in the back, Linda crouched in the hatch and Cassandra drove while I sat shotgun. We passed by and through mountain ranges with exotic names like Sierra del la Porsima and Sierra Madre de Oriental while Spanish love songs wept from the radio. About two hours past Monclova we finished cutting through a magnificent mountain range and spat right onto a monstrous plain, with one gash running straight through, highway 57, our home for the next two days. It's here that I'm most at peace. There's nowhere else I'd rather be than on the road, stretching over beautiful landscapes and tearing toward some destination with a purpose. "There's nowhere else I'd rather be than right here," I quietly told Cassandra. She smiled back at me.

In the next eight days we rode all the way down to the southwestern tip of Mexico, lost Dan and Linda, Junior suffered a split chin, Cassandra suffered a severe urinary tract infection, all of this as we scrambled through the cities of San Miguel de Allende, Saltillo, and Morelia, along with the towns Real De Cotorce and Zihuatanejo. It sounds awful, but it was actually a wonderful adventure.

The calculated risk had paid off. Anytime I'm around Lobo I'm aware that he can blow the whole thing up in a fit of irrational rage at any moment. We'd come close there for a second. The simple act of being around him involves an unspoken wager that he, and only he, can tame the beast inside himself to a controlled froth. Every now and again he can get away from himself and stumble over some triviality, unleashing a well of negativity that festers inside him, a well that balances out the gregarious waterfall we know and love him to be. Like all bets, you can't win every time. The odds are usually stacked toward a favorable outcome, but nevertheless, he's as predictable as a newly domesticated animal, a temperamental child, or an aggravated genius, and can turn on you in a whim of his own perception.

Discipline

Lyme taught me discipline. In the months prior to my diagnosis I found a level of discipline over my thoughts that I never knew I had. Over the course of a month I learned to carefully monitor my thoughts and expel all doubts, precisely at a moment when doubt is all that reason would have me focus on. After my diagnosis I had to tap into a different form of discipline. With the diagnosis coming after nearly three years of searching I felt that I owed it to myself to take full advantage of the second chance I'd been blessed with. That meant going sober—cold turkey—no easy task for someone that hadn't been sober for a day in a five-year span and whose entire social network thrived on inebriation. I wondered if I'd need a new set of friends, though that question was instantly put on the back burner. All that mattered was making the most of the opportunity to be healthy.

Every night during the first several months of sobriety I kept having the most vivid recurring dream where I was surrounded by a group of friends and someone would hand me a joint and I would suck it down greedily. Every detail of the dream flashed in my mind with stunning clarity when I woke up and I would curse myself for being weak and giving in to temptation. I would stumble to the shower giving myself a pep talk about how I had to be stronger, and that one slip up wasn't the end of the world, but this could never happen again. Then halfway through my shower I would pause and realize, *wait a second, I was just hanging out alone last night, no one came over, I haven't seen my friends in years.* Then I would laugh at my foolishness, only to repeat the exact process the next morning. These dreams faded away with time.

At this point I haven't touched a drink or any drugs in eleven years. Sobriety is a discipline that Lyme demands from me, and one that's still a challenge today. The social pressures of drinking to be able to fall into the same frame of mind of those around me, particularly with a new group of people, is a prevalent force. Being around a crew of drunk people is like trying to laugh at an inside joke, but the best I can do is smile because everyone else is laughing.

There's also some internal thirst that rears its head once in a while and cries out for gratification. Once in Mexico, seven years into my sobriety, Lobo and I were driving along the coast when he hopped out of the car to go talk to someone. He handed me the 24-ounce beer he was drinking as I waited in the car. Instantly I could almost taste the Corona's cool, refreshing fizz trickling down my throat. My mouth felt drier than it ever had and the bottle began to be drawn up to my face, as if my lips were magnetized and the bottle made of metal. The beer felt heavier than lead and lighter than air at the same time and as I looked at it I could taste it, taste the drunkenness, taste the way I would sink back into the seat with a swirling buzz to my thoughts if I downed the whole thing in one go. The bottle became too heavy for me to hold, I had to drink it or put it down, and I quickly shoved it under a shirt on the floor. When Lobo came back in I told him, "Drink your God damned beer before I pour it out on the fucking street."

"Don't have to tell me twice," he smiled, and took a slug as we sped off.

Moments like these arise less and less as more time transpires. Today I barely remember what it's like to be high, drunk or tripping, outside of the fact that it felt good, outside of the fact that there was a release of tension, and a stumbling in step with mobs and madness. Today I've accepted my place outside the culture of inebriation. If I go see some music, I quietly sip water as the joint sways in drunkenness. I've accepted my spot on the periphery as an observer of the wildness at the rare parties that I do attend, and only occasionally does a whiff of a joint make my eyes grow big. And when my eyes light up in that way I just gently lower them to a calm level and continue on my way. The discipline comes in accepting that sobriety is the only way things can work at the moment and deciding before the beer is placed in my hand, before the smoke tickles my nostrils, that I'm going to turn it away. That way there is no hoping for the best and there is no decision to make on the spot, because the decision has already been made.

In February of 2008 I sprained my back in an attempt to make it back onto the court after a nearly three year layoff. That layoff began when my legs started to ache again in 2005. From 1998 to 2008 I had been able to play basketball for two years, 2003 and 2004. That fact hurt me. Even in the best case, a basketball player is given a finite number of years he can play, and I was eager to go out enjoy what games I had left in my body. The clock was ticking. Pretty much most of my athletic prime had slipped away; I was thirty and had spent most of the last decade watching from the sidelines as my body struggled with the musculoskeletal symptoms of Chronic Lyme disease. But around the end of 2007 my legs began to feel a lot better and I prepared for my second come back onto the court. My first several attempts went pretty well, but I was always remarkably fatigued afterwards, so I should have known that something wasn't quite right, that the disease still had a hold on my body and by exerting myself at such a high level on the court I was giving Chronic Lyme an opportunity to gain some ground in the constant battle between bacteria and immune system.

But I was in no mood to heed early warning signals. In February of 2008 I was feeling good. I was fresh off a beautiful trip down south where I visited Lobo and met his uncle in the Texas borderland. My body had performed well on the trip. I drove long hours alone, slept in the back of my car on a frigid winter night, and generally kept pace with all the craziness a trip with the De Los Reyes clan comes with. I had been doing push-ups and pull-ups every other day for nearly three years as I waited for my legs to stop aching. Finally, I felt I was ready.

The third time I played I realized I was wrong. Early in the first game I caught a pass on the wing, took two hard dribbles to the left, then planted my right foot and jumped back into a fade away 15-footer. I felt it right away, a stabbing twinge in my lower back. I felt the violent spasm before I landed and I knew right then that the pain was back, and would be back for a long time. I limped off the court nearly doubled over in pain and couldn't get out of bed for nearly a week. When I returned to work, I returned in pain, delicately maneuvering through the workday with my lower back in the forefront of my mind at all times.

After several months the pain had become more manageable, though it would flare up into something excruciating at least once a week. I tried employing all I'd learned from the two-month experiment seven years prior, but the faith was forced. I couldn't find any peace in it. I told myself all the things I'd said in the past, "I have faith in God, I will be healthy," but I couldn't find the right rhythm, I wanted it too much. At times I got angry at the pain. Other times I would beg and reason with God. I tried to find that patient, persevering attitude that had carried me through the worst of times in the end of 2000, but fell into frustration and disbelief instead. I wasn't prepared for a major setback.

In the spring of 2008 I decided to move to Austin, setback or no setback. That summer I packed my car, and, determined to make a trip out of the move, drove north to Wyoming, then south to Arizona, and finally east into Austin.

Ten days after leaving DC I was in a campsite outside of Sedona, Arizona. My back had tightened up badly several times already on the trip and I could feel a flare up coming, though I did my best to ignore the warning signals and enjoy the road like I had the previous two summers. I woke up before dawn to a sharp spasm in my lower back. I tried to roll around on my mat and find a position that alleviated some of the pain, but I found no relief. A dull, tight ache radiated out from the acute twinge in the center of my back. Each inhale sent a stabbing sensation up the entire breadth of my back. Chronic pain is a lonely, lonely thing when you're far away from home. A heavy sadness draped itself inside of me, and my heart deflated like a balloon with a leak.

I stared out at the stars through the mesh screen of the tent. It should have been an inspiring vision, but everything I saw and heard ran through a filter of physical pain and discomfort, and so this beautiful sight filled me with grief because I felt I was being robbed of an opportunity to enjoy it properly. How could this be happening again? All I could think of was how tired I was of being in pain, how it almost felt ridiculous that I should have to face this challenge again. Hadn't I already conquered these demons in 2000 and 2001? I couldn't do this again. Why was this happening? It was too much of a burden to ask me to start over again, I had grown so accustomed to the relative health I enjoyed in 2006–2007.

Mentally and emotionally drained I did the only thing I could think of, I began to pray. *I have faith in God, I will be healthy. I am loved by God, I am going to be healthy, I have faith in...* The words fell hollow and dead out of my mind. They were worthless. In disbelief I continued to recite my lines. I didn't know what else to do, I didn't know what else to say. I kept at it in a near panic, as I got sadder and more desperate with each repetition. Could anyone even hear me? Had I been fooling myself all along? How could this pain really be back in my life again? Why was there no power behind these magical words that had meant so much to me in the past? I wanted immediate results. I wanted a lightness in my being to fill my chest the instant those words entered my mind. I wanted to know that things would be all right, the way I had known at the end of 2000. I got nothing.

Sleep never came. The birds began to sing and the first glow of dawn crept over the horizon. It meant nothing to me, the whole morning was dead to me because I hurt too much to notice it. And that made me just as sad as the pain because I knew I had lost something beautiful and powerful over the years. The kid who, nearly eight years ago, had basked in the benefits of the two-month experiment, who could smile as he trudged through the rain and all his body ached, that kid was dead. I wanted to scream and pound the ground, but I could barely move. I lay there and took one shallow breath after another, grasping for something, anything. *I have faith in God, I am going to be healthy. I have faith...* My back shuddered in pain and I wondered how I would get up, how I would keep going. I was in the middle of Arizona and still needed to drive through New Mexico and Texas. *I have faith in God. I am going to be healthy.* I felt empty and defeated, and lonelier than I had in nearly a decade. Faith had become a crutch for me, a means to an end, but I wasn't ready to admit that because I didn't know what else to do.

I gutted it out for the next two days until the flare up subsided and the pain returned to a more tolerable level. Four days later I was in Austin, back in college for the first time in ten years, working in a new pre-school, and beginning what appeared to be a new chapter in my life. But it was more of the same. I had to learn how to deal with chronic pain again.

Dancing While Standing Still
April 2009 and May 2010

"For as the body is one, and hath many members,
and all the members of that one body,
being many, are one body: so also is Christ."
—The Holy Bible, King James Version, 1 Corinthians 12:12

Lobo and I were tromping around Austin once again. I'd moved down a couple of months back, bought an old RV, and parked it in his yard. The best of our travels together were behind us, having occurred in a two-year stretch where I'd felt relatively strong. Things had been falling apart within my body for over a year, and I was due to bottom out several weeks later. A band we had been told we shouldn't miss was playing downtown and we were primed to go.

The club was packed with people before we got there. A line turned around the block to get into the place. I had no idea a bluegrass band could draw this kind of crowd. They weren't exactly a bluegrass band, but a representative of a new sound flourishing in the northwest. This new breed of bluegrass crossed the folksy banjo roots of the old timers with improvisational, jam-band type explorations.

My back hurt before we left Lobo's house. My back had been hurting for a steady year at that point. I immediately realized that finding a place to sit down would be a pipe dream. It took me about ten minutes, but I managed to carve out a spot for myself along the bar rail at the very back of the club, right behind the slender avenue of space where the packed crowd allowed people to shuffle back and forth to the bathroom. I leaned on the bar and rested my aching back the best I could. Bodies constantly pressed up against me to slide past, clumsily stepping on my feet in the process. I held onto this spot dearly. Standing up for more than several minutes without some form of relief constricted the muscles in my back into a set of knots pulling against each other. I breathed and tried to release the tension from my back through a heavy exhale. It would work for a moment, a split second of release, but before I could inhale again, the pain would be right back.

The band was incredible and moved the entire audience. They had a fiddle player, a banjo, mandolin, and a couple of guitarists, along with a tight rhythm section. And their singer was gold, a young buck that sounded like he'd been plucked from the Appalachian Mountains 100 years ago. I leaned in the back and tried to enjoy it the best I could. I closed my eyes and focused on the sound, heard the sound with my whole body, like a wave rushing over and through me. The fiddle got to me. For a moment I felt as if the music coming from the fiddle was leaping off the stage, soaring into the air in a giant, neon arc, and nose-diving into my soul. A dance floor spontaneously formed at the base of the stage, a mass of people writhing in unison to the music. The music moved me too, and I wanted nothing more than to run up and join them. I felt a great pull within me to leave my spot by the bar rail and meld into them. Pain radiated out from the center of my lower back, up coils that pulled at my sides, begging me, demanding that I sit down that very minute. I get exhausted thinking about it. I clung to the bar rail.

Lobo's face popped in and out of the crowded darkness. He was slamming down one drink after another. His eyes burst with madness. I knew mine looked tired. I could feel them drearily sinking into my skull. At one point the music grabbed him and he hurled himself into the dance floor and spun around in this timeless, foot stomping, waltz. He was lost in the music and the moment. He was drunk out of his mind, dancing, clapping and stomping because the music told him to. I felt like that once, in Chicago, a couple of years back.

I saw Lobo spinning in the center of the dance floor and he seemed to create a vortex, like the whole club was made of water and he was a drain that someone had just pulled the plug from. For a second I was pulled up from the bar rail. For a second I leaned forward instead of back, but I immediately felt a pinch above my tailbone, and remembered the throb that hadn't left for a year, and eased on back against the rail. Lobo kept spinning, clapping his hands and stomping his boots with his head bowed down and his eyes tightly shut, as if they were just too lit up, as if his eyes might pop right out of their sockets if he didn't squeeze them closed.

I didn't move. I ached to, but my back ached more, so I stayed where I was. I watched Lobo form a tiny circle out of the mass. Somehow it made me feel better to see someone living it up. My pain didn't decrease, it just didn't matter as much anymore because even though I couldn't dance, he could. As long as someone was dancing, truly dancing with passion, and fervor, and fluidity, my soul could rest in peace. He captivated me out there for a second. I was looking so hard I almost placed myself in his shoes, felt the floor pound against my boot as he stomped his feet, and my hands thud into each other as he clapped, and the music whip me around like I was a puppet as he spun in circles. If I looked hard enough I could put myself in there from my stance on the bar rail. You can mark this spot on that other time line I told you about, the hidden one.

I started to realize that I didn't need to completely, physically immerse myself in every situation I was in to enjoy the moment. I lost the pressing need to feel and absorb all the physical and emotional sensations of an experience for myself. All the things I yearned to feel with and on my body, all the things I wanted to feel with my mind and soul, I could feel through others. I learned to look at people, observe their faces, feel their vibrations, peer down into them and almost place myself within their consciousness, thereby experiencing life as they do with my mind. This sounds less intense because I'm living on the periphery of the action, but it can be even more intense because you can gain access to multiple perspectives at once, particularly in a large crowd.

More than a year later I was at Barton Springs, this swimming hole that's found a way to live in the center of Austin, and there was a full moon concert by the pool. The headaches were limiting me on this evening—the type of headache that I have to focus on my breath to move through. There was a band set up by the diving board and a hoard of people surrounding them, packed in the tight, concentric circles. Every several minutes someone would arch their neck and howl at the moon, starting a massive communal howl from the group. I watched people howling and felt the rush of wind charging through their throats. I walked up to the edge of the mass and peered into the center. I watched them all. I felt the rhythm of the dancers. Next to them a young girl gripped her mother's hand, wide eyed in wonderment and slightly overwhelmed, but also secure because she had her mom. I felt it all through her eyes. I glanced over at a couple embracing at the edge and felt the love they had for each other at that moment. I could feel the tunnel vision that possessed them and only allowed them to focus on each other. I saw the moonlight blend in with the spotlights of the pool, casting oblong shadows in all sorts of angles. The late summer breeze swept in and ran over my shoulders. I ran with it. I became a keen sensing machine. I still hurt, but I didn't focus on it because I was more than just my body, I could touch all of it, the entire evening.

There was no their experience and mine, there was only one, the experience and the observer melding into one. For a second I breached the separation of all our constricting egos and lived as the experience of the pool on a full moon. Maybe that's part of the point that the mystics seem to harp on, the recurring theme that our separate lives are an illusion. Taoist sage Chuang Tzu insists that "nothing can be seen as other." I've run into that concept several times and I started to get a vague outline of the concept, like that tingling feeling that runs through your brain when you've almost figured out how to go about solving a riddle. I'm sure there's more to it than this, particularly because I can't exactly tell you what "it" is, but the quote from Allan Watts, "it is seen that the separation of thinker from thought, the knower from the known, the subject from the object, is purely abstract," did seem to ring a little clearer that night.

Walter Strikes Again
July 2, 2007

Being docked for two days, the itch to break open the road and point ourselves somewhere new grew and so we left Crater Lake, driving through the evergreen wilderness of Oregon, on a mission to find swimming holes along the Rogue River. Driving the rental still felt like somewhat of a betrayal, but the Honda was gone, and I had all but moved on. Costa and I had waited around the Bay area for some kind of news about the car for nearly a week. Everyone roundly told me that if I didn't hear anything about the Honda after several days, she was as good as gone.

A white Ford Focus was our ride now. A rental. No deep bond to anchor myself to—just a piece of metal on four rubber wheels. Nonetheless we were off and feeling pretty good. Somewhere on the California-Oregon line we had left the sour taste of car theft to float away in the Smith River. We came upon Jacksonville, Oregon where Walter, the colossal fuck up from the Big Lebowski, and Costa's Oakland alter ego, was destined to strike again. Jacksonville lies twenty miles west of Medford. It's a small town with a swanky, upscale country vibe about it. "Looking good Jacksonville," I said, raising an impressed eyebrow. "They got their shit together here, Costa. A little lacking in character, a little forced maybe, but no fucking strip mall sprawl, that's for sure." A sign read 'free meat, cheese and wine tasting'. I was hungry. The peanut butter and banana sandwiches on the menu for lunch today could wait in lieu of this exciting news of free meat and cheese. "We gotta stop," I told Costa and I saw his eyes light up with the prospect. But when the sign led to a gourmet restaurant/grocery store Costa got cold feet.

"I don't know, man, I don't think we should go in, we look like animals." I had to admit we were a grisly pair. My hair was beginning to feel and look like steel wool, my jeans were torn and stained with baked beans and fire soot. Costa didn't look much better. Nevertheless, free gourmet meats and cheeses are not something to be turned away, so I insisted. "Come on Costa, are you serious, it says free meats and cheeses, let's go," I chastised him, pushing him past his embarrassment and into the store.

There were free samples everywhere. At first I went around and sampled the entire circuit, then narrowed my scope and indulged in my favorites. I especially liked the buffalo sausage, practically clearing out the plate they'd left on the stand. I'd eat several pieces, walk two steps then turn around and walk right back, pretending to stumble upon this new and interesting buffalo sausage. Each time I would shove four or five pieces in my mouth, then leave to repeat the whole process all over again. By the time we left I was a satisfied, bloated mess. As we left I yelled in a panic, "We need bread," which we did, pointing to the grocery store across the street. It was here that Walter emerged from the shadows inside Costa, as he turned the corner way too hard and ran over the curve at full speed. I'm referring to Costa's Oakland alter ego, Walter Sobchak, the affable sidekick from The Big Lebowski who can't seem to get anything right and has a knack for complicating his friend's plans with his blunders. When I got out of the car I heard the back right tire hissing like a snake and knew that Walter Demas had fucked the rest of the afternoon.

Costa responded to the hissing tire deflating before us with the meek, disbelieving look I thought we'd left in Oakland. After we lost the Honda a great wave of doubt overtook Costa. His usual self assured cockiness shrank away and he agonized over every decision, seemingly running his thoughts through the gauntlet of all that could go wrong if we turned left at the light, or went to eat at four instead of six. It was actually comical, especially since it was opposite of what I was used to seeing from him. His brown eyes, now all sad and puppy like, had some mixture of kid lost his candy and deer caught in a land of headlights look about them. The strut had completely crumbled from their midst and bore no resemblance to the coy, playfully sharp eyes, that held enough twinkling arrogance to make you root against him in small matters. I knew Jack in particular would revel in this new, uncertain Costa. "Come on. Come on," I moaned to the sky, throwing my hands in the air exasperated. "What the fuck, you really channeled your inner Walter this time Costa."

"I'm sorry, man," Costa said quietly as I walked into the store to buy the bread and let him deal with putting on the donut, the whole time shaking my head at the slap stick futility of our incompetence. We drove twenty miles back to Medford with all our belongings stacked on the sidewalk by a Wal-Mart oil and tire center. Three hours later we had a new tire and were ready to continue south to the beloved Smith River. "It's funny the momentum of life and how little things can run you off course," Costa reflected as he drove.

"Yeah, it's a powerful, yet fragile thing," I answered.

"A couple of things go wrong and you lose your confidence, or at least part of it..."

"The part that lets you act without doubt," I said, finishing his sentence.

"Yes, exactly. Well," Costa drew to a conclusion, "it's a fine dance on the line, not everyone can do it," implying he was one of the few that could. The balls on this guy. The last three hours roasting in the sun all because he cut a corner way too hard and still cocky as a God damned rooster. This grated me and ill sentiments resurfaced from two nights past when for some forgotten reason he had gotten on my nerves and I was rooting for the mosquitoes to bite him, inwardly smiling every time he wailed about another bite. I started to wish a locust of mosquitoes would swarm through the vents and accost him. The image of him screaming, attempting to swat them away in vain as they mercilessly fell upon him like a school of piranhas, put a vindictive smirk on my face. If there was any justice in this world those vents would explode with a locust of mosquitoes, the cocky, arrogant, stupid son of a bitch would be brought down a peg or two then, that's for sure.

Playing My Song
April 3, 2009

*T*en years after I first fell into the blues, I slouched onto the couch in my RV, picked up the cheap resonator guitar I'd bought after Oakland got my first one, and started noodling around. Four years ago, spring of 2005, marked the first time I picked up a guitar. Lyme disease put the guitar in my hand.

By April of 2005 my legs had just begun to hurt again. At that point I'd been playing basketball again for a little over two years, and thought I was home free of the disease for life. Giving up the sport for the second time hurt me because I loved it. Basketball was a spot in life where I felt that my creative source could find expression in a way that was perfectly suited for me. I loved the exertion, and the flow of the game, and the way I could get lost in the rhythm of the sport and find myself in a mindless, meditative zone—where my body reacted within the confines of the rules. But that was all gone again. All of a sudden I had this huge chunk of time, but even more importantly energy, that I used to devote to the court, free and unspoken for.

After waiting five months for the pain to subside, I bought a guitar. I was unsure if I could teach myself to play at the late age of 27, but was determined to give it a try. In the late 1990s, before my diagnosis, I had been too sick to try and learn the instrument; holding my body over the guitar would have been excruciating, so I had given up the idea then. Once I got healthy, I devoted every spare moment to basketball because I'd missed it so badly for five years. Now seemed like the perfect time to learn. My legs hurt all day, ruling out sports, but my upper body was in nowhere near the poor condition that it was in 1999. It took me several months to play a chord cleanly and six months to write my first song, but now, five years later, I can't imagine my life without a guitar in it.

I looked out of the RV window and started playing. Suddenly a new riff—a new song—jumped off my fingers. I didn't plan it. I had a slide on the pinkie of my left hand, and the fingers of my right hand just kind of found a rhythm, spontaneously building a song. My left hand, with the brass slide, glided up and down the neck at the 12 bar blues timing and chord progressions, and my right fingers picked my steady song. Excitement doesn't begin to describe what I felt. I was clicking like an intricate, soulful metronome—right on time. I was plugged into some hidden source of creativity, and the sounds I created rained into my ears, cascading onto the excitement that possessed me and fueling it further. The whole thing seemed to continually build upon itself. The more I heard myself, the more intensely I played. I thumped my country blues for an hour straight without realizing. I played my nameless song until my fingers were blistered and raw. When I stopped I put the guitar between my legs and rested my brow on its head. The last hour bounced around inside me like one long, euphoric echo. "Thank you," I whispered. I was talking to the guitar, and maybe whatever creative spirit had been flowing through me, but I should have been talking to the disease. The disease put the guitar in my hand in the first place. Ain't life a trip.

Leave No One Behind
August 13–September 9, 2007

I'd left Lobo and the rest of the De Los Reyes crew in Austin several days ago. The summer of 2007 had proven to be a wild one. I lost the Honda out in Oakland in June, then flew down to Austin and drove all through Mexico with Lobo and family in July. Our trek through Mexico ended with one mad sprint back to Austin, which left me dizzy with exhaustion afterwards. It was now mid-August and I was back in DC, fresh off the flight home and pondering just what to do with the $6,000 check the insurance company had awarded me for the stolen vehicle. I'm slightly ashamed to admit that after more than a month I had written the Honda off and was lustily eyeing a used Toyota Tacoma pick up with an extended cab and a cap for the bed. During mid muse I received a phone call from officer David Richard of the San Pablo police force, asking me if I knew an Anthony Love, if there was any reason why he, (Tony Love), would be driving the Honda. For a second I mistook the name for Tubby's and said, sure I know him, I stayed with him in Oakland. "Really?" The officer asked me in a stunned voice.

"Oh no, that wasn't his name, never mind, sorry," I muttered.

"Yeah, I didn't think you'd know him, Love's kind of a street creature," Richard told me in an official tone, as if his words were filling out a report in mid air. *Tony Love=Street Creature, Nick Vittas=Suburban theft victim, conflicting pieces of a puzzle that shouldn't fit. All is well.*

I was told that the car looked fine, that even the factory radio was still in place on the dash, so basically Tony Love had taken the car on a six week, 2,500-mile joy ride. I felt a little pang of guilt for writing the car off the way I had. How could I have forgotten that the Honda is no ordinary car, that there is a little magic moving her pistons? Wasn't she the car that amassed 17,000 miles the previous summer? Wasn't she the angel that had carried me safely on all my travels so far? Me and that car have breathed life into each other over countless miles and landscapes, with company or in solitude. Through all the unpredictable turns that all trips naturally take, the Honda was always the one thing I could count on. What she lacked in style and traveler's comforts she more than made up in a steadfast, almost mystical, reliability. And now, after six weeks away she had found her way back to me, making a long distance call for one more trip out west before the summer died. I knew I had to go out and get her. Only a butcher could sever such a strong tie with an enchanted little shit box like that, even if there was a sizable check on the other side. And on top of everything, my loyalty would be rewarded with a dash across the continent. How perfect. I had three weeks to pull it off before work started again in September.

The next day I got less that rave reviews for my loyal ideals. My parents, cousins, friends and co-workers all roundly proclaimed that I was a sentimental idiot who was taking a grave risk by retrieving a car that a thief had used and abused for nearly six weeks. *Who knows what he did to that car in that time? It will leave you stranded 3,000 miles from home and you'll have thrown away the insurance check for a car that's destined for the junkyard. Use your head. These are childish notions*, and so on and so forth. Only Costa was onboard for the retrieval mission. Costa saw the larger picture, the beautiful, mad poetry of riding the Honda triumphantly back across the country, of completing the trip as originally conceived in early June—before car theft was a thing I automatically associated with Oakland—of the final adventure that was attached to the whole thing and the chance for our own slice of redemption with the road, and the car, and the Bay area in general.

When I called the insurance company the next day I was surprised to find out that returning a claim check is a lot harder than I expected. I figured they'd jump at the chance to get their $6,000 back for an 11 year-old heap, but they were actually stonewalling me. Apparently once the claim goes through, the title has switched hands, and the check is in the mail, the process is irreversible. I tried to find every loophole imaginable, even suggesting that they tell me which auction block the Honda was destined for so I could buy it from whichever salvage dealer bought her. All I got for my efforts was a bunch of "Sorry Mr. Vittas," "There's nothing we can do Mr. Vittas," "It just doesn't work that way Mr. Vittas." Finally I simply asked the agent to look into it and see what she could do.

I was with a friend the next day, touring second hand music stores for an affordable guitar, when I got a call from the insurance company that washed away any doubts that the Honda was indeed shrouded in an orphic aura. Due to a clerical error the final step of the paperwork, where the title is sent to the DMV and the transfer of ownership is finalized in the government's eyes, was never completed. Since the transaction never reached this point of no return the door was open for me to give back the check and retrieve the car. I immediately called

Costa and started bellowing into his voicemail, "the Honda's back baby. I always said she was a magical car, and due to a clerical error, a fucking clerical error, I'm getting her back. Stop pretending like you have something better to do, I know you don't have a job, pack your bags and get on board, we're bringing the Honda back."

During the next week Costa and I just loafed around his apartment and the neighborhood bars and coffee houses, and the week dragged by slowly. Progress with the Honda moved slowly too. It took three days to drive the certified check over to the insurance company and get the title back, and another three days to orchestrate the Honda's transfer from an impound lot to a mechanic in Fremont, California. Costa had lost his job upon returning from Oakland and had a big interview scheduled for the 28th of August. He was a nervous wreck about it. I had my own problems to deal with. Tony Love did a real number on the Honda, totaling $1,800 worth of damages to the underbelly of the car. I spent my afternoon putting on my best adult face and swapping phone calls between the mechanic in Fremont, California and the insurance company who I'd just handed back a $6,000 check. In the end the insurance company said they'd cover everything, though they made me sweat for it. There were a couple of hours in between where I thought the bill was going to be laid on my lap, like a loyalty tax.

At the end of the week Costa left for the interview looking sharp in a freshly pressed suit and just enough desperation to show he meant business. If he got the job he'd ask to start in two weeks and come out with me to retrieve the Honda. Without a job he would have to pass on the adventure. He seemed optimistically nervous when he returned. "How'd it go?" I asked him.

"I don't know, man. I think it went pretty well. The director said she's not one to mess around and that she'll give me her decision within the next 24 hours. I need this job, Niko. I need this one," he said, gripping my arm and howling at the ceiling. "I looked over at this paper she was marking during the interview. Most of my answers she had marked down as fours, I think out of fives. That's good right?"

"Sure," I shrugged. What did I know; I walked in and filled out applications for jobs. I'd yet to fill out a resume, much less have an interview.

We were at my parents' house the next day when Costa got the call; he'd landed the job. We were going. We ran to the basement and started fingering routes across the map. As best, and loosely, as we could plan, we would pick up the car in Fremont California, continue north to Portland, then up to Seattle, jump the border for a quick hello to Vancouver, per the original, pre-theft plan, and then zip back across to DC, back in time for my work, which began on the 10th of September. We counted days and approximated miles with giddy disbelief—just how much could we fit into nine days? "This is unbelievable. This is so unbelievable," Costa exclaimed. His eyes were aglow with anticipation. He'd been bitten by the bug, if only temporarily, and the concept of heaving himself across the country in a hurried, mad dash not only seemed like a wonderful opportunity, but a necessity, a fix. I eyed the map like it was a feast, and became hungrier by the moment.

Two days later we were in the San Jose airport, en route to the dealership where the Honda awaited. We had left Costa's apartment at four in the morning in an attempt to grab the car and make some real headway north into Oregon that same day. The attempt was made in vain.

There was some mix up with parts and the car wasn't ready until right before the dealership closed at seven. We got the car as they were closing. The wheel was oddly crooked, resting at three o'clock instead of completely level and the keyhole was missing from the gearshift. A big empty hole remained from where some blunt tool had been used to pry it off. I went to plug in the ipod and immediately noticed the cigarette lighter was broken. A slight panic rippled through my chest. Within twenty miles of the shop the "check engine" blinked on, and the rippling panic was now a tidal wave smashing every rational thought from my head. *Fuck.* This car not only had to make it back home, I had to get at least three more years out of her or else I'd never hear the end of it from the long line of naysayers who had begged me to take the check and leave the car out west. *Fuck. Every time I want to do some dumb fuck thing that makes no sense, this car will be rubbed in my face*, I thought to myself. *Fuck. I should have just taken the money.* I kept my worries silent and quietly begged the car to act right and make it home until Costa noticed the "check engine" light and demanded we take stronger action than wishful thinking. We decided to get a room near the dealership and have the car looked at as early as possible the next day, since the present one had slipped away from us. Hopefully we'd be on the road by noon tomorrow.

By the time we found a cheap motel it was nearly eleven. The radio had blown out as we pulled into the parking lot. I pushed all the buttons in frustration but nothing happened. At this rate we would need to be towed back to DC before we got out of California. There was a Denny's next door and I ordered the meat lover's breakfast. It was a plate of eggs surrounded by the cheapest, greasiest meats available: bacon, sausage paddies, kielbasa, and a steak of country fried ham. "Why'd you order that?' Costa asked as he grimaced at the heap of grease and flesh on my plate.

"Just you know, because, 'fuck this'," I quietly snarled back.

"What does that mean? What does that have to do with that disgusting meal?"

"I don't know Costa, it just seemed appropriate, that's all. Don't ask me questions I can't answer," and I went ahead and cleared my plate with contempt. We ate in bleary-eyed silence. Back in the room I was asleep before Costa turned the TV on.

Costa and I were at the doors of the dealership when they opened at seven the next morning, and within two hours found that the radio was dead because of an easily replaceable blown fuse, there was no way to replace the cigarette lighter that day, they didn't know why the steering wheel was crooked, but it drove straight so we were told not to worry about it, and the check engine light had "just come on for no reason." We escaped for the road immediately, balling north on 101 with golden, honey painted hills rising around us, a working radio in the dashboard, and a real pep in our step.

We clipped past the canopy of tunnels the Redwoods create, past the spot where we dropped off Powerful, Puffer Fish Ron, past Eureka, and Crescent City, pushing hard for the Oregon line. Something was different about the handling of the car. I had to ease off the gas a lot more than I used to when turning a corner or else the back would fishtail, as if we were skating on ice. "What was that?" Costa asked me as the car jerked to the left rounding a turn.

"I don't know. It's weird, right?" My brow furrowed as all the unspoken pressures of the Honda's rescue began to mount again. My God damned reputation was married to this car now. The engine purred as soft and beautiful as she always had, but the handling was off. What had Tony Love done to this car? What misadventures had the Honda been in with that thug? More likely than not, with 2,500 miles added on by Mr. Love, the Honda was probably a drug running mule. Another momentary slip around a turn brought an uneasy grin on Costa's round face. "Fuck it," I told him, "She'll be fine." There was really nothing to do about it at this point other than to take the turns a little slower than usual and keep rolling along.

Oh, but I did feel wonderful to be back in the Honda again, fishtailing or not. We put the old girl straight to the test, 700 miles in 14 hours, and wouldn't you know she responded marvelously. I was supremely comfortable behind the wheel. With each passing mile I felt my soul being sewn more deeply into the fabric of the car. Nothing could fit me better. The imprint of my body lay on her seats, and the imprint of my soul lay on top of hers. She's my darling. With one hand loosely gripped on the wheel I was in my own bubble of righteousness. This is where I belonged, in this 11-year old shit box. We shot like an arrow straight through the night, (except for the occasional turn when the arrow would wobble), all the way to Portland. There we spent a night with one of Costa's flings from way back in high school. The next day we left her and went off to Seattle for lunch on the pier.

A quick lunch and we bounded north again, continuing to Vancouver. A strange and wonderful sense of accomplishment rose in me upon the realization that we were actually completing the trip as originally planned. The pavement hummed in harmony with the Honda. The evergreen vastness blurred by as mountains shot up and down. The car would occasionally fishtail, particularly around turns, but perhaps this was her post theft limp, a little scar from the road. I was a little uneasy about her new condition, but realized there was nothing else to do at this point other than put a little faith in my girl and keep going. She'd gotten us this far, hadn't she?

We came upon Vancouver and I winked at the city with a trivial sense of closure. Take that Tony Love—we finally made it. Costa had another girl waiting for him in Vancouver. That guy never ceases to amaze. By morning we were finally marking our route east as we peddled to Canadian Highway 3. Vancouver quickly became a smaller and smaller cluster of slender buildings behind us, shrouded in overcast skies, looking like concrete fingers stretching to tickle the clouds. The city vanished in the rearview mirror and my heart trembled and throbbed at the magnificent sight of the great North Cascade Mountains ahead, and our sacred Highway 3 slithering right through. As we continued, rugged mountains began to ascend around us, mountains that are breathtaking and strike at the bell of your soul, announcing the beauty of God, and life, and art, in an unmistakable ring that resounds silently throughout you.

The Rolling Stones' "Let it Bleed" sang from the radio, blasting at maximum volume to overcome the wind roaring in from the windows. It was the album of the trip, a group of songs that now seemed to be perfectly in step with the journey, the car, and the changing surroundings. Each trip naturally develops an album like this, one that slowly builds momentum until that's all you want to hear, your own personal soundtrack of the road.

As we shot east, the sun burned away the overcast skies and spread itself blissfully on my arm. I was back in the Honda, back in my little black cannon ball, shooting across the land at seventy miles an hour, as everyone—me, Costa, the Honda—burned to go. I danced in my seat as my right hand gripped the wheel and my left hung out the window. My head spun around and my eyes sharply focused on everything, intent on ingesting every last detail. I drove this way, feverishly, yet effortlessly, a witness as much as a driver, for the better part of the next ten hours. It was marvelous.

I pushed us through the North Cascades and toward the Monashee range. We labored over an arching incline, and there, to my surprise, exploded a vast fold of copper hills, cascading down like yellow falls of the earth. Green trees and grey boulders peppered the scene. Costa dozed in and out of consciousness, paying dearly for his night of excess in the city. The drive became even more wondrous as we continued, like something out of a picture book, a fairly tale of the great, beautiful west. These were the drives I left home for. These are the drives that, as Lobo muttered in Mexico a month prior, "Fill your being."

Crystalline waters delicately wove a path through the mountains. At one point we pulled the car off the two-lane, asphalt ribbon highway, over to a little bridge that connected two dirt roads. We leapt off the bridge, into the cold cradle of the river for a quick swim. Then back to the car, eastbound. The sun fell in the rearview. In the mountains of British Columbia, darkness falls like a black velvet sheet draped over everything except the slivers of white cut by the car's headlights. We called it a night on the border at Grand Fork.

In the morning we crossed the border and balled through Washington's sagebrush desert, over Idaho's panhandle, and into Montana. The scents of Montana blew in from the open windows: a combination of cowboys and cattle, and the wild, vast freedom of open prairies so grand your spirit called to leap out of your constricted body and stretch and soar in their space. We were making great time. If we were lucky we would get to crash in Chicago for a night of blues before returning to DC, and work, by Monday.

We clipped right, off I-90, onto highway 89. After gliding through prairies and plains all day long, the Rockies were back. Their dark, jagged peaks pierced the clouds above. A river, the Yellowstone I believe, snaked along the highway and through the mountains like a great, dark reptile. Light was quietly leaving day. We had all but resigned ourselves to the fate of riding through the night until we came across some motel somewhere, until Costa spotted a tent on the banks of the river. He immediately U-turned the car and within minutes we were in the most beautiful, most serene, most majestic roadside campsite I'd ever seen. The dark river, smooth and fast, drifted by not ten feet from our tent. Across the banks the Rockies stoically towered over us, running north into Canada and south into Wyoming and Colorado. They were so large and close that it seemed I could reach out and touch them, and so sharp they carved a vivid, black separation in the grey, overcast horizon. Yellow grass and slender, arching trees blessed the embankments. I'd never seen anything so perfect in all my life.

Remarkably there were only two people there aside from us, an elderly couple. The husband was fly-fishing in the last remnants of light as the wife patiently waited. They soon left, leaving the whole scene to us. In all our wildest dreams and prayers of car campsites we never could have imagined anything so uniformly perfect. We set the tent up under a little grove of trees, door facing the mountains. I could hear the dark water glide by in the still, silent night. I swam in place within the strong current of the river. We ate our dinner of chili and bread by the banks as a strange night glow offered just enough light so we could make out the shadows of the mountains looming in the darkness and the sweeping, liquid lines of the river dashing by. As far as I was concerned this was a gift from the Honda; she was the one that brought us out here.

In the morning the dawn light glittered off the river. Birds chirped and gossiped and sang in the trees as fish acrobatically leapt for their breakfast. Great planks of light burst through the clouds, shining heavenly spotlights on the dark green hillside that crept up to the mountains. Amidst the beauty, Costa noticed that the outer half of the Honda's right rear tire was almost completely worn down. It was feathering badly. The tread had totally vanished and the tire looked as if it could blow at any minute. We had to backtrack an hour to Livingston to get it changed. "The alignment's not fucked up, but something's clearly not right back there. You feel it sliding on all the tight turns, right?" I asked. He nodded. I felt Chicago slipping away from me. *Come on Honda, you've made it this far, don't pull any shit now.*

Two hours later we were on our way again as the first pellets, of what would prove to be a torrential downpour, began to drop. We'd gotten lucky in Livingston, finding an open shop with a short line. "Something's peelin' that baby off," the mechanic commented on the worn tire, "no way of knowing what unless I put her on the lift and take a look. Booked up today, though." We replaced the tire and cut out as fast as we could. Hopefully the new tire would last until we got back to DC.

I'd been driving no more than an hour when the sky broke open and torrents of rain whipped down in furious, incessant lashes. I buckled down, nose to the steering wheel, and strained to find the road within the blistering storm. Trucks roared by, several feet from us in the opposite lane of traffic, kicking up great waves of mist that splattered against the windshield. I hunched over the steering wheel even more, searching for the road between the frantic slashes of my windshield wipers. Every couple of minutes the Honda would fishtail and briefly hydroplane on the old, slick highway, which had a thick film of water constantly streaming over it. Each time this happened I had to ease off the gas, and gently, but firmly, guide the wheels back under control. Costa begged me to pull over. "I'm not comfortable," he screamed, "Just pull over and wait this rain out."

"We'll be fine, we'll be fine," I tried to console him as we swerved again and I had to quickly gain control of the car.

"Did you feel that? We're hydroplaning, Niko. Pull over, please. I'm not comfortable." He repeated this last part many times, but I brushed him off and kept right on going.

I drove with the fiercest focus I could muster, and put every ounce of my being and will into sharply concentrating on every crevice of the road, seen and felt. I channeled my inner Lobo; everyone has a beast like that roaming in their depths. I was vehemently determined to continue, and to continue unscathed. A quick, violent swerve shook us both, and Costa began his pleading protests again. "Look Costa, we can't stop because it's raining. What if it rains all day? What if it rains tomorrow? We gotta get back to DC in three days and we're in Wyoming. And we're trying to stop by Chicago, no?" I pushed on through the rain, fishtails, and protests.

"At least slow down, go fifty Niko. Please, for me as a favor, go fifty." I conceded, as the fishtailing was getting stronger and wilder and harder to control. I knew something was wrong with the car. This is not how a normal car responds to the rain. My eyes scowled and blazed like a demon's as I peered low and looked through the tiny pocket of visibility that my beaten windshield wipers offered. Some monster within me drove. I would have been too scared to go on. I could never drive so fiercely. I felt as if only the most bare aspects of my mind existed. I found a rhythm of intense determination and relaxed...comfort. It was attune to those moments back when I could play basketball where I'd fall into the zone and hurl contested, fade away jump shots—jump shots people defined as 'prayers,' but I knew the ball was gonna fall right through the rim, even though I couldn't see the hoop, and only verified the fact that the shot had dropped true by the sweet sound of the net swishing back and the disgusted reaction of the man guarding me. It may sound stupid to make such an analogy because one deals with a game, and the other with real life ramifications; but like I said, my inner Lobo was channeled. We were going to make it to Chicago, God damn it; the blues was waiting for me there. "We'll be fine, we'll be fine," I said after each swerve and on we went as Costa muttered prayers and curses.

The rain subsided later that night and we stopped well into morning, somewhere in South Dakota. As sun up spoke its motel slang—cars starting, janitor's trolley squeaking—I basked in the remnants of a wonderful dream. It was a vivid dream, where everything I'd seen from British Columbia through Wyoming slid by like a movie, except I saw it from the air, like a bird. Every mountain, canyon, lake, and prairie glided by in pristine detail, and somehow time sped up so I flew over all that we'd driven over in the past days in one night, in one resplendent dream. All the colors: the greens, and yellows, and blues, leapt up at me in the sky, and when I woke up I had the most extraordinary sensation of living the last few days twice. We found Chicago the night after that, and then home after that.

As it turned out, when we got back to DC we discovered that the rear right control arm was badly damaged, and this was the cause of all our unsettling fishtailing. How the mechanics in Fremont missed this last souvenir from Tony Love I have no idea, but apparently we were in some real danger out there. Somehow the magic Honda delivered us home safely, and with one more adventure to marvel at under our belts. After all the criticism I got for taking the risk to go fetch her a week prior, she had performed remarkably, cranking out an eight day, 4,500 mile journey just like old times. This trip galvanized my image of the Honda as an unshakable, faithful companion. So far I've taken the car on eight more trips, averaging around 3,000 miles each way, with nary a problem. Tony Love gave her back to me with 120,000 miles, and we're well past 200K and going strong as I write these words. Sometimes I think there's a little shaman that lives in her guts, quietly and dutifully fixing things before they go wrong, keeping us on track, and always on the go. She's a little slice of destiny, an eight ball that always finds a way to glide straight into the right pocket eventually. My little, black cannon ball. The Honda.

To Be Coated and Immersed
April 2010–October 2010

"When we accept what *is* without avoidance,
we will find there comes a state of being in which all strife ceases."
—Krisnamurti

I had a hard day at work. I knew it was going to be tough before I even left home. I felt the muscles behind my neck and on the sides of my head tighten as I ate breakfast and I could tell things would only get worse from there. Within an hour my head throbbed, and kept banging for the rest of the day. As the eight hour shift progressed the pain spread from the back of my head, crawling like a spider out across my temples, digging its fingers into my cheeks and eye sockets. At times I hurt so bad I couldn't see right, my vision took on this distorted, black light contrast.

I didn't quit and go home. I gutted it out, delicately pushing on, wary not to plow ahead and bring on a full collapse, but also persistently sticking to the duties of my job. Shuffling along through eight hours at the daycare, I took care of my kids, breaking up fights and settling squabbles, setting up art projects and offering encouragement, all in a more subdued manner than usual, but I got the job done. The pain yanked on my head as if someone had screwed the muscles under my scalp into a tight knot converging at the top of my neck. I didn't have the energy to think about anything else other than whatever activity with the children I was engaged in. Each moment of the day demanded my complete attention because the pain I had to sift through left room for little else. Thinking of the past would have crippled me. Pondering the future would have swept the rug from under my feet. Even lamenting on how hard moving through the day in pain is would have added another burden to my already depleted energy reserves. I dealt only with the immediate task at hand. And thus I stumbled onto a judgeless state, where immersing myself in the "gutting-it-out" mentality brought me into a meditative trance of endurance. I had nothing left when I got home. I ate a quick dinner, laid quietly in the flickering glow of the TV and drifted into sleep.

Several days later I was driving home listening to Co-op talk radio. The guest was a lady who had started an organization that used ponies as therapy for people suffering with all sorts of emotional and physical ailments. This lady had been through a lot herself. She had been raped. She had been homeless while caring for two young children. She had battled breast cancer for years, losing both her breasts, and now suffered through chronic pain as a result. The DJ was nearly bowled over by the list of hardships his guest had endured. He asked her how she could cope with so much adversity, and the lady answered, "in each instance I asked 'what am I supposed to learn here? Help me learn it as fast as possible so I can take the exam and move on.'" Those words resonated with me. What was there for me to learn from my experience with chronic pain? Curiously, I had never directly asked that question despite the fact that I was consciously aware of all the ways the illness had humbled and enlightened me along the way, prodding me to evolve into what I considered a better and more well rounded person.

I examined the mentality I'd fallen into at work the previous day. It was one that had been slowly materializing for some time, but now I took a closer look. Was this "gutting-it-out" mindset somehow connected to a lesson I could benefit from learning? If so, what could that lesson be? The value of keeping one's mind in the present moment had appeared in several texts that I had been reading, particularly Krisnamurti. This view of living completely in the *now* did seem to directly correlate to the frame of mind my thought fell into when the pain was worst, when I had to gut-it-out. When the pain was the strongest I would lose the energy to judge the situation as positive or negative, hard or easy, fair or unfair. Instead I focused all my energy on moving through the present.

Days and weeks after hearing the broadcast the notion kept growing in my head. What could I learn from the disease? Often when a part of my body would flare up in pain I'd ask myself what was there to learn from the situation—though I didn't always finish the thought, the question had begun to arise. Six months later my back happened to flare up in particularly intense spasms. Pain radiated from the center of my lower back, over my hips, rolling up under my ribs. The flesh on my sides trembled. The message seemed to crackle through my whole body—we're in misery. I was at home, in the RV. I lay down, closed my eyes and tried to find the rhythm of my breath. The question popped in my head, *what can I can learn from this sensation running through my back?* I asked myself again and again until somewhere in my mind I made a partial detachment from my body—I had a body, but there was more to me than my body, I was the observer of the body's sensation, the asker of the question. I wasn't my back, but the observer of its sensations. I took a step back and watched the pain without branding it in a positive or negative light. I observed the pain that shot its way through my body like a dull, electric surge. I observed it from within and from a distance, sympathetic but strangely unfazed. None of the hurt from the past thirteen years registered. It didn't pile up on me like it sometimes can because I was only observing what existed in that moment.

This moment is all there is. There is no reason to think of any moment other than this one. There is no reason to think of possible future hardship, because it does not exist now. Making it right now and living right now is all there is, and I am making it. That is all that counts. I'm not worried about how I will walk around tomorrow if this spasm in my back doesn't die down, how I will take notes in class, study for my exam, go to work. None of that exists now. I'm not tired from years of the same muscles aching in the same ways. That happened then. Only what exists now is relevant. I'm breathing in my bed. My belly is expanding and retracting. There is pain behind it but I just watch it. I don't loathe or fear the hurt. I don't put a judgment on it as a negative trial to endure. I register the sensation of pain shooting through my back along with the ceiling fan's currents caressing my skin, and the crickets' layered rhythms of chirping rolling in through the open window. I am the observer of all these things—so I simply observed the way all these vibrations registered against my body. I was coated in the moment.

There was no need to scheme and reason and conjure up ways to change my future into something more desirable, so this weight was dropped from my mind. The past was wiped clean by each passing fraction of a second, and could not weigh upon me either. All that was left was the present. The peace associated with this slight change in mindset went past the days when my body ached the worst. On days that I felt fine there was no point in worrying about the headache that lay waiting around the next corner, or wondering how long it would be before I could work out again if I kept feeling good. Neither of those possibilities existed *now* so I let them go.

Planting myself firmly in the present made an impact on me beyond my physical health and how I reacted to parts of my body flaring up. I started to realize how often my mind aimlessly chattered no matter how I was feeling in regards to Lyme. I saw that I spent a large part of my days rambling in senseless circles of 'what if's' and 'could be's'. I began to quiet these internal dialogues and observe my surroundings. The internal silence brought the beauty of the ordinary and mundane sharply into focus to the point where I could sit alone in a packed dining hall and notice that the cafeteria's buzz sounded like an orchestra, and the more I'd listen the louder the symphony of voices and silverware and trays would get until I'd almost get knocked over by the shear intensity of the sound. I didn't always remember to see things in this clear way, but a little pinch in the back or at the back of my head would remind me, and I'd sit back down into the present.

One thing didn't sit right with me though: there was a contradiction between firmly planting myself in the moment and the faith that had started my journey ten years ago, the faith from the two month experiment which was based on the notion that ultimately I would regain health. Was I to completely abandon my goal of health in order to stay in the present? Was complete passive acceptance of what *is* the only way to connect with peace? This contradiction aside, I did feel happier when I tuned into the moment, and so I let the contradiction stand on its own, unsure what, if any, resolution would arise.

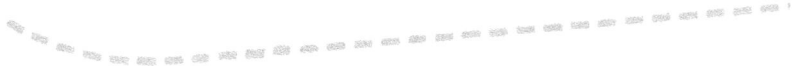

Love and Exhaustion at the Mexican Flea Market
August 3–10, 2007

Cassandra, Lobo, Junior, and I rolled in from our ten-day tour of Mexico short two Americans. All six of us had crammed into Lobo and Cassandra's Toyota Matrix for the ride down, but somewhere in the Pacific beach town of Zihuatanejo we'd lost Dan and Linda. They'd opted to separate from the group for a romantic night alone and we were never able to meet up with them again. Truth be told the insides of that car were getting so cramped that there had been no real urgency on our part to find them. Stuffing six humans into a compact Toyota is no easy task. I wasn't too worried; they were both resourceful and would surely make their way back soon.

Junior was sporting a fresh set of stitches from where he split his chin at the beach. He actually split his chin on his mother's forehead as a wave crashed down on both of them. Cassandra was nearly doubled over in pain, by what we later found out was a weeklong urinary tract infection, while Lobo had been on the grind to get back to La Madrid by the 3rd of August and spend some time with his little sister who had traveled all the way down from Nebraska to see him, his son and their mother. To arrive any later would mean battling bombardments of guilt trips. He was already in the hole for neglecting to visit her after her hip surgery in the spring. She was still recovering from that now, walking around with a slight limp. It all stemmed from a car accident she had in the winter of 1998, which actually coincided with the seizure that sent me tail spinning down the road of illness and recovery as well. If nothing else, Kayla and I had always shared the bond of lost health and the pain of seeing the world freely roll by as some part of our bodies was broken and wouldn't heal.

Kayla had been waiting for her brother in La Madrid for two days by the time the tired and battered carload of travelers pulled into the driveway of Alejandra's house. Kayla's husband had stayed behind in Nebraska, unable to secure any time off. Alejandra is Lobo and Kayla's mother. Both Alejandra and Kayla are small thin women, dark and athletic. To look at Kayla is to see Alejandra twenty some years ago, and to see Alejandra is to peer into Kayla's future. They have lean faces with large round cheekbones cupping dark, round eyes. Both ladies immediately gushed over Junior as he bravely displayed his battle wounds from the road. They took turns pressing the three-year old boy's head to their breast and grieving to the Virgin Mary for the thin scar beneath his chin.

The porch was cluttered with a mass of junk, looking like a yard sale that had been plowed through by a tornado. Alejandra had collected all this stuff from yard sales in the states, rummaging through her own possessions, and grabbing the occasional item deemed unnecessary from her family members too. It was Thursday night, we were to sell all this stuff at the flea market in the nearby city of Monclova on the weekend with the unspoken, but widely understood notion that the proceeds would be put directly toward Alejandra's truck payment due several days ago. Lobo's father had run off to the Dominican Republic a few months back. She had rented out rooms to make up the mortgage, but was on her own for the rest of the bills. This was as good a plan as any, I guess.

By the time morning broke the next day Kayla and Cassandra had already left for the clinic in the town over. They'd be gone all day. After breakfast Alejandra took her grandson to play with his cousins down the street. Lobo started to work on the stove, which had a leak that stank up the kitchen with gas anytime it was turned on. It started to rain, softly at first, then quickly building to a splintering fervor. The roof leaked in five or six places, three of them quite heavily. I scampered around with buckets and pots, placing them under the leaks as fast as I could. They rhythmically tocked like a sad drum as Lobo crouched behind the stove, rubbing soapy water on the pipes to try and spot the leak. Eventually he found it, took the pipe apart, then taped it shut best he could. The smallest pots had to be dumped out before they overflowed as the downpour continued. The pool outside, ten feet deep aside from the section Lobo filled with concrete in an attempt to make a baby pool, (which by the way dropped straight into the perilous deep), had four feet of murky water and algae crawling up its walls. A lame mesh fence that protected no one from falling in ran around its borders. The house looked good, but disrepair was creeping in. Alejandra would sob about it later in the night, storming off to conceal her tears, leaving Kayla anxious with guilt. Lobo, as always, cracked jokes. As long as he isn't upset, anything and everything is a joke to him. It's all fodder to be mocked and exposed as inconsequential in the grand scheme of life's varied and complex brilliance. His jokes proclaim that life's cosmic absurdity and soulful humility are the true things to get worked up about. In some regards it's his greatest character trait and greatest personality flaw too. These jokes are perfect, and reveal people's grievances for the petty, trivial gripes that they are. On the other hand, it does seem a little hypocritical when he can't see his own peeves in that light, but a mirror can blind even the best vision. "Man, Dad is off in the D.R., slapping some bongos with some big brown bitch, having a good time," he said, tapping an imaginary set of drums, "and I gotta deal with this shit." He motioned to the door his mother had just run out of. As always it was delivered at precisely the moment of strongest tension, right when Alejandra slammed the door on her way out. We all laughed. Even guilt ridden Kayla couldn't help but crack a smile, because in the end it really all is funny.

After the storm cleared Lobo and I started to lethargically file through the junk his mother wanted us to sell the next day. We weren't really doing anything, just taking stock of what was there and sometimes moving a heavy item closer to the truck. Lobo wandered off to the edge of the yard. He bent over pensively for a couple of minutes then spun around and broke into a sprint straight at the pool. He let out a victorious cry, a wail from the depths of his crazy soul, and leapt over the mesh fence, flipping in mid air and landing in a tucked cannonball, splashing dirty water up over the ledge. He bounced up and thrashed around in the water, slapping, punching, screaming, as he disappeared in the froth. When he was finished he climbed out with a tremendously self-satisfied grin plastered on his villainous, dark face. Water dripped from his drenched clothes as he sloshed his way to a hammock. We were supposed to organize, price, and pack all the junk. We did nothing. It would be the last moment of idle rest for nearly a week as things became so frantically busy there was scarcely a moment to breathe, and sleep turned into a desperate commodity to be scratched out in whatever dark hours remained before dawn. It all ended disastrously as I collapsed from exhaustion on Alejandra's living room floor in San Antonio five days later.

I passed out on the couch. Halfway through the night I awoke with the unshakable intuition that I wasn't alone in the living room. I lay in the dark and laughed nervously at myself. It was the second time I'd been steamrolled by the fear of seeing a ghost or being seen by a ghost in this village. Try as I might I couldn't calm myself in the dark so I turned on the lamp by the couch. I'd heard so many stories of ghosts from so many different people that it seemed the land here was sowed with so much emotion that spirits sprouted from the ground like corn. Perhaps Alejandra's ghost would haunt the land she had cried over long after she was dead and gone. With the light on I fell asleep. An hour later I woke up to darkness. Muttering timid curses I flipped the switch back on and fell back asleep. Several hours later I awoke to a dark room again. What the hell was going on? Was the lamp fucking with me or what? "Hello, is anyone there?" It was Kayla, apparently as scared as I was, talking to the darkness in the middle of the night. She had been the one turning off the lamp, as the light slipping into her bedroom fell on her eyes. On top of anything supernatural that may have been going on we were haunting each other, turning lights on and off behind the other's back. We had a good laugh at our foolishness. "You're scared of ghosts?" she asked in disbelief with a twinkle.

"That's two summers in a row that ghost shit has gotten into my head out here," I told her. We both agreed that there was something different about the land in La Madrid.

"It's why I've been sleeping with my door open," she admitted.

The alarms were set for six in the morning and obnoxiously went off on time. Alejandra was up. Kayla was up. Lobo was certainly up, pacing in and out of the house. "Vittas, you gotta help me load up the truck," he called as he blew past me on the couch and onto the deck. I groaned as I got out of bed, did some quick stretches and joined him out on the porch where mounds of junk lay. A more random assortment of shit never existed: trash bags of clothes, mystery bags and crates filled with anything from crayons to toasters on the top layers, (and even more surprises stuffed inside), heavy table saws, chain saws, VCRs, book shelves, gutted AC units, working AC units, a plastic lawn table and a set of chairs, and countless other nick-knacks, all of which we painstakingly loaded into the truck in a massive heap tied down nonchalantly with a single rope. The whole process took forty-five minutes and immediately after we finished Lobo got in the truck and revved the motor; it was go time. Alejandra chuckled as she watched me inhale a bowl of oatmeal as I ran to the door. No one else had the foresight to eat anything.

And it was here that we were merriest, with some urgent, pressing, matter driving us somewhere, anywhere. There was a buzz to the manic energy of the process and the careless sarcastic jokes about the whole thing. We could enjoy it, unfazed by the pressure, we laughed while we sped 80 miles per hour with a truck load of God knows what shit, to sell to God knows what people, and needing to make 500 dollars over the next two days. Cassandra and Kayla drove in front of us two in the truck. Cassandra waved her hand for Lobo to pass. "What is that?" he desperately asked, "Is it food?"

"No, it's not food, you fucking retard," I barked back.

"Oh my God, I'm so hungry I'm going to piss someone off just so they'll punch me in the face and I can eat their hand," Lobo moaned. We laughed uproariously as if we were high, and in a sense we were.

The hour drive to Monclova went by quickly in this way. Cassandra, the pearl of Monclova, led us to the flea market where we bought two plots for nine dollars apiece. The girls would have one plot for all the clothes and shoes and related accessories and Lobo and I would man one for everything else. There had been concern on the way that we wouldn't find a spot, but apparently we were an entire day early. The handful of merchants there informed us that Sunday was the major day of business. No matter, we were already there and the plots were paid for, so we set the whole gamut up in a mad scramble. Lobo and I unloaded the truck again. We had a canopy that went over the girls' plot. They hung clothes from hangers on the crossbeams and arranged shoes, purses, and the "cheaper" clothes neatly on a blanket beneath the white tent. Lobo and I spread a large blue tarp over our plot and started to dig through the many crates and bags that lay between the larger items such as table saws, heaters, fans, chainsaws, and VCRs.

The things we found in those mystery bags and crates you wouldn't believe. The full spectrum of the beaten, second hand human experience lay in a cluster upon that tarp. A crate of note books and one of crayons, a sealed pack of depends, a cat food dish, binoculars, jump ropes, VHS movies, DVDs, a broken Fossil watch, barbies, an electric massage pillow, coffee makers, lamps, drills, pliers, coolers, tupperware, two new bottles of shampoo, an old laptop, stuffed animals, TV trays, comforters, a toilet seat, dismantled fan motors and their assorted parts, mugs, salad tossers, a cell phone with the box and charger, a battered, ancient, camera, tool boxes, and much, much more. Passersby would come up looking at us, and our whole operation, with suspicious curiosity. Who were these eccentric fellows, with this absurd collection of junk, changing prices, inventing prices on the fly, bickering with each other in English, then quoting a whole new price. It was almost like a circus sideshow and even though the market was pretty dead that day we drew the most people to our site.

Kayla and Lobo answered questions and pushed for sales with frenetic zeal, electrified by the environment and the opportunity to stand center stage in their very own auctioneer show. Cassandra rested in the shade, still weak from her infection, while I hovered around trying to make myself as useful as possible, straightening out the chaos of our derelict wares and occasionally selling an item in my broken Spanish. All the money went into a change purse that Cassandra held and I ran back and forth making change between the two camps. The purse got fatter and fatter throughout the day; we were actually selling a fair amount of this junk. It was well past midday, the Mexican sun belted down upon us as if someone was holding it an inch from our heads, and we suddenly realized how rabidly hungry we were. Cassandra was sent off to get some tacos, and remove herself from the sun in the process. Just as she was leaving this massive woman, donned in spandex shorts that seemed ready to split and a sports bra that accentuated the considerable rolls of fat stacked upon her sides, came up to Kayla and started bartering over a pair of shoes.

The pace slowed down in our camp and so Lobo and I sat back in our lawn chairs, (which were for sale), and watched this cow of a woman work Kayla over. She had short hair and her front teeth were capped in gold. She smiled at Kayla like a well seasoned thief as she amassed a great number of clothes, got a price quoted, then had Kayla add it up again with the intent purpose of trying to fool her into either lowering the price on an item or forgetting to add it to the total sum. The whole process repeated itself many times. The cow brought great bundles of stuff to Kayla, then after everything was added and settled upon she would ask, with an innocent smile, how much this shirt or those shoes were again. Kayla would have to rack her memory for the price she'd made up, and since there were no price tags the cow would naturally protest that Kayla was mistaken and the price of this shirt or those shoes had been half that. "Now let's add it again," the cow would smugly suggest. Kayla became more exasperated with each cycle and started calling out numbers for us to remember, drawing us into the whole affair.

Lobo and I started to root for Kayla like she was involved in some grand sporting event. "Let her have it Kayla," I screamed.

"Give it right back to her, babe," Lobo roared.

"Kayla, Kayla, Kayla…" we both chanted in the background. All we needed was popcorn to go with our front row seats. The cow and Kayla went at it for well over an hour. It was all great fun and the cow played the villain wonderfully, shooting a sly smile our way when we got particularly noisy.

"Where the fuck is that woman with my Gat damn food?" Lobo gripped. I shrugged my shoulders, Cassandra had been gone for a good while. "Is this some kind of sick, sick joke," he continued, "it's almost like people HAVEN'T not eaten all day."

"I don't know what to tell you Bo," I offered, but he persisted, constantly grumbling his disgruntled comments.

"This must be some kind of sick fucking joke," and then several minutes later, "Vittas, just tell me, are you in on this sick joke?"

"What do you think Lobo, Cassandra's hiding in the bushes, passing me fucking tacos every time you turn around."

"All I know is that this has to be some kind of sick joke," was all he could answer.

"Chinga Madre," we suddenly heard Kayla shriek, throwing her hands in the air then shoving money back into the cow's hands. Her gold-capped teeth flashed in feigned innocence while Lobo and I howled and hooted, applauding from our tarp. The cow relented, having the gamesmanship to know when she'd pushed her opponent too far, she tried to give Kayla the money back while clutching the clothes she'd always intended on buying. Kayla refused it at first, but it was 180 pesos, eighteen bucks, and we didn't have the luxury of refusing big-ticket sales like that, so in the end she had to accept the cash.

Cassandra arrived right when the cow was leaving. "She's still here," she said in amazement.

"Never mind that," Lobo blurted, "where the fuck have you been?" Cassandra explained that the first store she wanted to go to was closed and so she had to drive further out. We attacked the tacos, wolfing them down ravenously, throwing four across the way to Kayla. After our late lunch we caught another rush of business. Kayla was distraught that the sparkling blue ballroom gown wasn't selling so she began to model it, the tail end dragging through the dusty gravel of the market. Amazingly that savage little princess sold the gown within half an hour, right off her skinny, little body. "They probably bought that for their daughter's middle school dance," I teased her. By four we'd been there a steady eight hours in the sun. Foot traffic had died down and the change purse was looking nice and fat so Lobo made the call to start packing up. He backed the truck up to our plots, we started to dismantle the canopy and the girls took over our tarp of assorted, derelict junk. A group of elderly women walked up and Kayla leapt into a fevered pitch to sell them a pack of new tampons. They resisted and Kayla hunched over, put her hand on her crouch and belligerently asked,

"What, you ladies don't get your periods anymore?" They were taken aback and quickly moved along, probably deeply offended by the petite girl with the filthy mouth who just made blatant references to the intimate processes of their old and withered vaginas. When Cassandra translated what just went down I nearly blew my top. I'd been riding Kayla for days about her savage tendencies, the way she sat or ate like a teenage boy or the crude things she sometimes said, but this one really took the cake.

"Why didn't you just say, 'what you bitches don't bleed from your pussies no more, what the fuck,' " I goaded her. The gall, the absolute raw savagery of her comment and the complimentary gesture was priceless and I loved her for it. She was a true savage princess and took all my jokes about it in good humor, with a cute, bashful smile, as if these crude, bestial things just popped out of her like a gaseous belch that slipped by her defenses.

Lobo and I loaded up the truck bed once more, this time with a considerably smaller amount of shit. I counted the money on the ride home, 2,000 pesos-that's 200 bucks on the slow day—morale was great. When we got home Lobo proudly presented Alejandra the cash and she accepted it nonchalantly, like a landlord collecting rent, but I could see through the modesty; she was pleased and touched by our efforts. All the money went into a small ceramic pot. It might as well have said "truck payments" on the side. Tomorrow we'd start all over again. Cassandra and Kayla went straight to sleep, enjoying a well-earned siesta. Lobo and I were draped upon the couches, about to do the same when I heard an ominous rumble from the sky. "Did you hear that," I asked.

"No," he lied. From the porch I saw a dark and determined sky looming from the east, one that you can almost see moving toward you.

"Shit. Bo we don't have much time, come on."

"Fuck," he grumbled, slowly rising to his feet, but when he saw the sky he sprang into action. I stayed by the truck and lifted everything out, either handing it to him or placing it on the edge of the porch. Lobo ran the stuff to the back of the porch, where it would be safe from the impending storm. We were hustling. The first droplets began to fall and we still had half the junk in the truck; if the storm broke open now it would all be ruined and turn from saleable junk to unsaleable trash. Our efforts doubled. We found a frantic rhythm of unloading, passing and storing until the truck was nearly empty. Right when I grabbed the last crate it was as if the black clouds, now directly overhead, were ripped open. A furious rain pelted down upon us, whipping through the swaying trees. I leaned against the porch and watched the whole spectacle unfold. It was quite an awesome storm, but only lasted for half an hour. It ended suddenly, like a switch turned it off. The sun burst through, and all the bushes and trees, adorned in droplets, sparkled in the light.

We all ate dinner quietly and separately. I was beat. The phone was perpetually ringing and a party was brewing at Alejandra's house. Some of Cassandra and Lobo's cousins from Satillo were on their way, along with the standard crew of local De Los Reyes relatives that popped by on a nightly basis. One of Cassandra's cousin's from her mother's side, Julia, had already arrived. She was a plump, mild woman with two daughters: one pudgy, Buddha looking eighteen month old and Himena, a sweet six year old. Himena had a beaming smile that radiated almost constantly and an angelic laugh that sang throughout the house as she and Junior ran and played.

Lobo had the impeccable timing of suggesting that we re-load the truck just as the sky became cloaked in darkness. "We wasted almost an hour packing this morning. Let's do it now and leave right away tomorrow morning." To further complicate matters Alejandra had been digging through the storage room in the back and discovered a whole new set of forgotten goods, (shit), that could be sacrificed to the sale, so we were right back where we'd started from in the morning. If anything there was more new stuff than shit we'd sold in the day. Back to the grind of packing that truck. This time we had to plan more efficiently because of all the new stuff Alejandra had added from the once cramped, now barren, storage room.

All the De Los Reyes family from La Madrid slowly started pouring into the house and were boisterously carrying on inside while Lobo and I painstakingly stowed everything back onto the truck bed in the warm, Mexican night. We kept getting interrupted though because the matriarch of the family, a great, bulky woman who took shit from no one and was the mayor of the village, had planted herself next to the fridge and looked badly upon drinking. Everyone except me drank but was too afraid to grab a cold one in front of her, and so came out to send me, a relative stranger, in to get it for them. I must have grabbed ten beers in front of her within a half an hour and if she was paying the least bit of attention I'm sure she was convinced I had a serious drinking problem. Lobo was included in this group that basically turned me into a living room bootlegger.

Halfway through the job Dan and Linda materialized into the porch lights like a phantom couple of the dark. They had made it all the way back from Zihuatanejo, bussing it to Morelia, then flying to Monterrey, and taking another bus to Monclova, and finally a bus to the village of La Madrid. We embraced quickly, then cracked back to work as they went inside to freshen up and lay their bags down. I found out later that Dan had proposed to Linda that first night away from us in Zihuatanejo. His bright blue eyes, set deeply in his meaty, boyish face, had a serious glow about them. Soon after they went inside the final carload of cousins arrived. One of the girls had a big, hulking, South African boyfriend who stuck out his big, meat hook hand to greet Lobo and was stunned when Lobo brushed it aside and leapt on him, grappling for footholds as he tried to reach the summit of his mountainous frame. The South African, who could have been a stunt double for Arnold Schwarzenegger, was naturally bewildered and froze for a second before throwing Lobo off. Lobo laughed manically at first, and then tapered off into a slow bobbing nod with a friendly grin. The South African cautiously put his guard down and Lobo immediately leapt for him again. This time the hulk was ready and just clobbered him to the ground. His girlfriend pulled him away, leading him toward the rest of her relatives in the house, but he glanced back several times to make sure the wild man wasn't rushing at him again. We finished packing the truck and made a quick prayer for no rain.

The girlfriend of the hulk brought one of her friends, a reasonably attractive, but somewhat bland girl, and all of Lobo's aunts immediately pounced on the opportunity to try and set me up with her. They were always devastated to hear that I was single and promptly took the most embarrassing route to introduce us, announcing publicly that we were both single. Thankfully the girl spoke no English and so I couldn't reasonably be expected to start anything with her, thus the whole awkward thing was over when the one aunt who spoke decent English, Cha-Cha, grew tired of translating.

I walked around back where Lobo and Dan were trying to light the barbeque. Someone had brought a mound of steaks and corn and Lobo had been charged with the responsibility of cooking it all. I was tired and fading fast. I just can't keep going nonstop like these guys. Even in my good years, and this was most certainly one of my strongest in a decade of chronic illness, my engine burns fuel faster than everyone else. I sat and listened to Linda and Dan recount their adventures while away from us, the best story being their stay in a hostel at Monterrey. The place was sleep in your clothes, on top of the sheets, filthy, completely unshowerable, and run by a bunch of drug addicts who left their weed scattered about the house. Everyone left for some mass camping trip, leaving the doors wide open, a sack of weed on the coffee table and Linda and Dan on the honor system. Their karma abiding souls didn't touch it. "What?" Lobo moaned, flabbergasted, "if that were me I would have smoked the whole fuckin' thing right there." Chances are that was true. The coals, meanwhile, stubbornly refused to light until Lobo found a can of kerosene and doused the whole thing with it, tossed a match, which nearly blew the old, rusty barbeque apart with the instantaneous explosion. "Those coals are cooking now, eh, eh?" Lobo boasted. I was tired and needed to sleep. The day had been an endless melee of action and effort and the prospect of staying up far into the night with all these people seemed impossible to me. Thank God my head didn't hurt or my back, those parts of my body would wane years later, and I could enjoy what madness my eyes could ingest while they had the energy to stay open.

The couch I'd been sleeping on was smack in the middle of the living room, surrounded by loud socializers and drinkers, but I noticed that Julia and Cassandra were putting Junior and Himena to sleep in one of the bedrooms. I seized the opportunity. "I'm sleeping in here on my mat," I told Cassandra and began setting up my camping mat at the foot of the twin beds. The camping mat intrigued Himena, her coffee colored eyes sparkled with curiosity. She asked her mother all sorts of questions and so I began to show her how it worked. After it was unrolled and inflated the sweet angel pushed me aside and began making my bed. After she'd tucked a sheet under the mat, neatly set a blanket on top, and fluffed the pillow, she turned to me with a pleased, glowing smile. "Gracias, gracias, que bueno," I applauded. Then it was lights out and I was asleep before either of the two young ones.

In the middle of the night I woke up. Cassandra and Junior were curled on one bed and Kayla was in the other. "Is that you?" Kayla drowsily asked. I answered her and asked what happened after I fell asleep around midnight. She began to ramble about some dance they'd gone to and all the late night talks with her cousins. I sat on the corner of her bed. She reached out and touched my forearm with her fingers, then quickly and suddenly jerked her hand away. I got up and went to the bathroom, almost certain that we'd both felt a sensitivity for the other in that touch, and positive that she'd abruptly snapped her hand back because that wasn't a path she wanted to cross as a married woman. I saw Lobo on the couch. He looked drunk even in sleep. He told me the next day that he'd stayed up hours after everyone else, drinking alone on the hammock until the mosquitoes drove him inside. Seeing him belligerently laid up on the couch gave me hope that we wouldn't be up before dawn the next morning.

My hopes were justified. I awoke of my own volition at the lavish hour of eight thirty, shortly before everyone else. A panic ensued and we scrambled to the truck with the fear that we may be out of a plot if we showed up at the flea market too late on the busy day. Again I was the only one who had the foresight to eat anything, wolfing down a bowl of cereal in thirty seconds as the horn blared outside. Lobo complained of hunger as we sped down the narrow highway with the truck loaded higher than the day before. When we arrived at the market it was too crowded to pull the truck up like we did the day before, so we parked on the street, against the fence. Our plot lay directly on the other side of the chain link fence.

Lobo, Cassandra, and Kayla ran over to the plots while Dan, Linda, and I unloaded the truck, lifting each item over the fence and handing it to Lobo who would place them on the tarp. Kayla and Cassandra tried to make some sense of the assorted junk piling up around him. We were late, every other vendor had been set up for hours and the market was a crowded, bustling conglomeration of bartering and transaction. Being late and thereby a fresh set of goods to assess, along with the unorthodox nature of our arrival, (passing each item over the fence in a human chain), coupled with the absolutely bizarre and universal scope of our wares, all combined to create a growing commotion. Sparked by curiosity that fed upon itself each time someone new gathered around the tarp, Lobo found himself surrounded by 20, then 30, and soon 40 to 50 people, each of them clamoring to see or bid on something. It was madness. People were bidding against each other in this shopping frenzy we'd unwittingly stirred up.

When the last of the heavy items had been passed over the fence I ran around and tried to weed my way through the crowd and onto the tarp. Theft was a concern, as well as the need to make some semblance of organization of the heap littered on the tarp. But even as I was shifting things around people were buying them right out of my hands. I left Lobo with Cassandra for a moment and organized Linda, Dan, Kayla, and myself on each end of the frame for the canopy— we pulled it apart and threw the tent over it. I ran to the truck and brought out the clothes, wrapped in a massive comforter that seemed ready to burst and plopped it under the canopy. Back to the blue tarp with Lobo, who was wheeling and dealing with no less than five people at a time. Cassandra and Kayla hastily set up their clothing boutique and took advantage of the run off sales from Lobo's tarp o' junk.

It was like this for over an hour and we sold an extraordinary amount of stuff. A young couple came up and started asking me questions about the laptop. I answered their questions as best I could in my broken Spanish and to my astonishment actually sold them the thing for 150 dollars. It was the biggest sale of the day. But right after the swelling glow of pride from the big sale died down I started to worry that the thing wouldn't work. I made silent prayers that it would. How awful to have swindled some poor, hard working family. "Relax bro, the thing works," Lobo assured me off handedly, which meant nothing. Cassandra told me that she's seen it used and it did work and this did put my concerns to rest. Linda and Dan had wandered off, Cassandra wanted to get the car detailed here in Monclova where it was cheap, and Lobo demanded food. The sensational pace of our entrance finally eased up and the purse was looking fatter than ever, (I mean shit, I put 150 bucks in there myself, bro.). Thus I left with Cassandra to bring back food and get the car detailed, despite the quiet oppositions of Lobo, who voiced concerns that the detailing would delay the arrival of his food.

"No, no," Cassandra assured him, "I'll get the car detailed while we're waiting for the tacos to be cooked."

Of course there were complications. The car detailing was going to take an hour and the taco shop next door had just run out of tacos for the afternoon. To further muddle matters, Cassandra ran into some cousins from her mother's side and we sat with them at the restaurant that had no tacos for the entire time the car was getting detailed. Tacos still had to be delivered to the hungry troops on the front line of the flea market and we sped the sparkly clean Matrix across town to one of the few taco shops open during the brutal afternoon hours when most shopkeepers and patrons have the good sense to siesta. The second taco joint took more than half an hour to deliver the goods, so by the time we headed back to the flea market we'd been gone for more than two hours.

"Do you think he'll be mad?" Cassandra asked me, biting her lower lip in consternation.

"He was getting there yesterday," I said, "things were becoming a sick, sick joke."

"Why is he so funny," Cassandra laughed. She was madly in love with him, but her laughter had a nervousness wrapped around it. To further agitate things, one of Cassandra's cousins had jumped in along with us. Lobo was not too fond of this cousin, Erika, and this would only serve to agitate matters further. When we finally got there Lobo was glowering at her with his arms crossed and sweat glistening on his face.

"Where the fuck have you been?" he bellowed, his voice projecting throughout the flea market. Cassandra's tender eyes dashed to the ground, hurt by her ogre-ish reception, but quickly bounded back up, staring off over his shoulder with indignation. Lobo carried on with a mean whip to his words. "It's not like I've been working all day in the sun with nothing to eat." She handed him the food then turned and walked away. He continued, louder now so she couldn't escape his voice. "You've been gone for eight hours. People are starving, working in the sun and where the fuck were you? Hanging out with your stupid cousins? Huh? Huh? Chinga Madre." Again I found myself in the position as the only one eating while the two of them were fighting over the preparation or deliverance of some meal. The same thing had happened down in Zihuatanejo, only that time Cassandra had been the slighted one when Lobo and I sauntered off and left her to cook dinner solo. I'd felt pretty bad after that blow up. This time I guiltlessly stuffed down the below average tacos, thinking to myself that Lobo was being utterly ridiculous. If he had really been that hungry he should have sent Kayla out to get one of those cheap street burgers while he watched over both camps. Cassandra held a grudge for the better part of two days, but as usual the ill sentiments between them blew over sooner than later.

Now we were all in the eye of their storm and their fight had sucked the wind out of our sails. We quietly and efficiently shut down shop and packed the truck one more time. When we finished loading up the truck the bed was only half full. Miraculously we had sold over half that junk off. What should have been a triumphant and jubilant moment was solemn and somewhat awkward. In the truck I counted the money in the purse as Lobo vented some more about Cassandra's gross inconsideration. There was 3,600 pesos—360 dollars. When we got home Lobo handed Alejandra the purse, with the money neatly arranged in one fat stack. She played it cool again, but I could tell she was pleased. Lobo recounted the madness of the first hour in rambling Spanish. And told her how I had been the one to sell the laptop. "Oh thank you, my Nieeeck," Alejandra said with warm, motherly eyes.

"De nada," I winked back. She wasn't the only one who could play it cool around here.

For the remainder of the day Cassandra walked away from Lobo as he followed her, trying to make things right, but withholding the outright apology that would. He took breaks every time a different door was slammed in his face, sitting on the porch and stewing about the whole thing. Despite my efforts he stubbornly refused to eat. "Come on Bo," I implored, "just eat some fucking tacos."

"I'm not hungry anymore," he somberly retorted. We had discussed driving to a swimming hole for a nice dip after the flea market, but Cassandra wouldn't go with Lobo and Lobo wouldn't go without Cassandra, so the refreshing dip was scratched. I lounged on the hammock and talked with Kayla. She made some fresh squeezed lemonade for us to sip on while we chatted. We had started to take care of each other in little ways like this: bringing a plate of food for the other, holding doors—I just naturally started carrying her bags and it seemed appropriate because who else was going to take care of her. Our conversation rolled on smoothly, seamlessly streaming from one tangent to another. Mostly we'd joke and she'd laugh as I picked on her savage, less than lady like, tendencies. Sometimes we'd lead ourselves to a serious topic and we'd speak softly in hushed voices and she'd lean close to whisper, but always careful not to lean too close.

Alejandra made a delicious dinner of mac n' cheese, handmade Mexican style. Cha-Cha came by and barraged me for not connecting with the girl from

Satillo the night before. "Nick, why didn't you do anything?"she asked in her thick accent.

"She was not good enuff for Nieeeck," Alejandra came to my defense. "Nieeck is the bes'. Es mi otro hijo." I blushed when I heard that. She said it sincerely and it meant a lot. After dinner we started to pack for our departure State side. Saidita, Alejandra's youngest sister who had married rich, had paid Alejandra 100 dollars to drive her and her three kids to San Antonio the next day. We were to leave by six thirty in the morning because her flight left San Antonio at three. Cassandra and Junior would ride in the truck with Saidita and Alejandra, the rest of us in the Matrix. Everyone's bags would go in the truck, which Lobo, Dan, and I had unloaded once again before dinner.

As I packed my bags in Lobo and Cassandra's room Kayla fluttered around me. I picked on her in the playful, off hand manner we'd grown accustomed to as I folded and crammed clothes into place. Cha-Cha stood in the doorway watching us, her round face, perched atop her round frame, tilted to the side. "Something is going on here," she declared to Lobo and Cassandra who were silently packing on the beds. "These two are like husband and wife the way they fight," she pondered in her heavy Spanish accent. Kayla's face turned red as she tried to laugh it off. "God forbid, if you ever get a divorce, this is the man you should marry," she finished, pointing her chubby finger at me. I shot Kayla an "I'm not so bad" shrug and she turned crimson red and left the room. Cha-Cha's closing comment was as much an indictment of Kayla's husband Dylan as it was a compliment to me. Dylan was a great guy, and treated Kayla like a queen, but he was as white as white can be. He came from a family of Omaha investment bankers and his value systems concerning money, chance, risk, social expression and repression couldn't be further from the De Los Reyes clan, who considered flying by the seat of their pants from one paycheck to the next a life philosophy and were used to elation and frustration being vented on an hourly basis. Due to this incredible culture gap, Dylan had a hard time finding common ground with Kayla's people, and therefore a hard time gaining acceptance.

I crashed on the couch as Jackie Chan movies blared from the TV with Lobo and Dan's howling outbursts stealing any semblance of sleep I could find. They finally let me be at one in the morning. Before the sun had cracked over the eastern mountains and before the roosters had considered attacking the day, Lobo was up and at it. To completely finish the process of stripping the once hopelessly cluttered storage room totally bare Lobo enlisted me to help him move a washer and dryer. They were both broken, but Lobo wanted to take them back to Austin and get them fixed so we stowed them at the back of the truck bed. He began carefully packing all the bags on the back of the truck, keeping intense diligence on the conservation of space. Saidita had married rich up in Boston and had developed overabundant, expensive tastes. We were warned that she had a sizable amount of luggage.

We got to Saidita's house before seven. She was a beautiful, well-kept, petite woman with a becoming, slender scar tracing down from her eyebrow to the bridge of her perky nose. She was in her late thirties, had given birth to three kids, but kept in great shape and could have been a Mexican model. She certainly had all the flare of one. She had that De Los Reyes slice of fire too. "Andale, andale," she yelled with a broad, gregarious smile when we pulled up. She was a firecracker, sparring with Lobo like a boxer while saying quick hellos to us and herding her children around. There were three more massive suitcases, along with several other smaller bags to fit into the shrinking space on the pickup bed. I had no idea they made suitcases that big, but somehow we managed to stuff them in. Lobo draped the blue tarp from the flea market over the heap of luggage and began the intricate and somewhat convoluted process of tying it all down. With a look of brimstone determination he scampered all over the truck, heaving mightily on the single rope that he weaved in inconceivable patterns through all the bags, the whole time beaming with confidence, like he'd spent years being trained in the most progressive and efficient ways to tie bags onto the bed of a pickup truck. We snapped some bungee cords over the heap for insurance and he walked around, inspecting the mess.

"Eh, eh?" he crowed, "That shit ain't goin' nowhere."

We raced up 57 toward the border. Lobo and Dan took the front seat of the Matrix, while Kayla, Linda and I sat comfortably in the back. There was scarcely a bag in the hatch, much less a human like on the ride down from Austin a month ago. Saidita roared the truck ahead and we followed. The tarp almost immediately became loose and flapped violently in the wind, tearing down the middle. We stopped at the first gas station, ripped it off and continued without one—that shit really wasn't going anywhere so the tarp was superfluous. Kayla sat between me and Linda and the effortless conversation between us sparked up again. In the cover of the roaring wind that charged through the open windows we were able to talk in relative privacy. I looked at her little brown hands and ignored a sudden impulse to grab one like she was mine. We were almost forced to act this way, forced to hatch something between us by the sheer dynamics of the group: Dan and Linda, Lobo and Cassandra, Nick and...Kayla.

When we crossed the border and left all the ridiculous stipulations on who could and couldn't legally drive the truck I offered to grab the wheel, partially to be helpful, but also craving to do a little highway driving myself. Alejandra and I switched vehicles. I hadn't been behind the wheel since arriving in Austin the previous month. Where art thou Honda, lost and forgotten in the Oakland night? I revved the truck's motor and we flew down the Texas desert plains. On the ride down Alejandra had plowed into a vulture with her truck. The massive bird had been picking at road kill and mistimed his flight, smashing into the windshield. The placing on the windshield where the vulture had been obliterated couldn't have been worse, directly in front of the driver. I struggled to look through and around shattered glass. I touched it and some tiny fragments of shattered glass rubbed off on my finger. It seemed if we hit a large butterfly the whole windshield would crumble and rush at my face.

As we approached San Antonio Lobo and the matrix veered off toward Alejandra's house while Cassandra directed me to the airport. I double parked the truck at the departures run off when we arrived and climbed up on the edge of the bed, hoisting each one of Saidita's massive suitcases up, balancing it on the edge while I jumped down, lifting them off the truck and gently setting them on the sidewalk. I did it three times over, and fast too, since I was blocking a lane of traffic. When all of her shit was finally out, Cassandra and I gave her a quick hug, then hopped back into the truck. I was panting in the passenger seat as we left.

We dropped off Junior and the Matrix in San Antonio with Alejandra and all crammed into the truck. Lobo wanted to get the washer and dryer checked out at a shop down the street from his apartment in Austin. The only hold up was that the truck was due back in San Antonio the next morning at ten to get the windshield replaced. Back to stuffing ourselves into tiny vehicle compartments, this time the cab of a truck. Well, at least it was an extended cab, still, no joy with massive Dan having to fold his shoulders to squeeze into the back seat with Linda, Kayla, and me.

There had been grave talk, (excited chatter for everyone else), about going out to the bars for Dan and Linda's last night in Austin, but I was all set and had been pushing real hard for a movie night and some well earned down time. As Kayla jumped in the shower Cassandra and Lobo fell sound asleep on their bed. Dan and Linda mopped around at the devastating sight of Lobo's slumber. Kayla came out of the shower all dolled up. Her hair was blown dried into a sleek style, she had a little make up on and she wore a fitted light blue shirt to go with her jeans. "Dang Kayla, looking good. Too bad you got dressed up for nothing more than a blockbuster night," I teased her motioning to her passed out brother.

"It's okay," she shrugged. She didn't really care. Dan and Linda were the devastated ones.

"You wanna hit the movie store?"

"Sure," she answered.

On the drive down there she was oddly silent, her tender face stared pensively through the shattered windshield. I felt something coming, and stayed quiet until it started to bubble to the surface. "What's happening here?' She asked in a quivering voice.

"I don't know." I told her.

"I feel drawn to you, but it's wrong, I love my husband," she fumbled along, blindly stammering. "Why didn't he come, I never would have talked to you so much if he had come." I just listened and said nothing as she rambled on about her guilt and shame for developing feelings for another man. And as I listened to her I began to feel flattered, and felt something that I'd barely noticed before, a great pull for her and her cute, effervescent madness. I guess it had been there since our first playful, teasings a week earlier, brewing and now it blossomed into recognition.

I should tell you that I fell for Kayla once before. But that was seven years ago. Back then Kayla and the rest of Lobo's family had come up to Amherst for Lobo's graduation from Umass. As it turned out he wasn't graduating, but he neglected to tell any of his family that, and somehow got his hands on a cap and gown and did the walk and everything. There was a big dinner in Lobo's fraudulent honor, and I was seated next to Kayla. We'd always had the bond of lost health, it's a connection you can't fake with someone, and so we started talking about faith and resilience in the face of a body that's not quite cooperating. After dinner, the partying in honor of Lobo's sham graduation began, ending far into the night with Kayla, Lobo, their younger brother, Bruno, and me watching a movie to shut it down. Lobo and Bruno almost immediately passed out on the floor, snoring in a drunken rhythm as Kayla and I sat on the couch. As soon as her brothers were out something changed in Kayla. She stretched her legs over my lap, her feet playfully rubbing against my crotch. I got up to get a drink. When I came back she was sitting, "you can lie down now," she told me, patting her thighs. I did what she said. Her fingers started tracing their way along my calves. Through all this I watched the movie with an unfaltering gaze. I couldn't look at her or stop her. She slid her way out from under my legs and lay down on top of me, resting her head on my chest as she faced the TV. My heart must have been drumming in her ear. Her fingers started to caress mine, and I gave up and caressed hers back. She propped her head up and dove in like a bird for a quick peck on my lips. And she laughed when she did this, as if it were so amusing. Then she dove in and kissed me again. Her brothers were right next to us. She was crazy. I kissed her back and her little tongue darted in and out of my mouth as I grabbed and squeezed her toned little body. Her brothers were right there; I was crazy. At one point she cupped my face and showered it with quick light kisses: my cheeks, my forehead, my temples, my closed eyes. It was intoxicating. The sun started to shoot through the blinds and Lobo began to rouse. She leapt off me, giggling at her madness. The next morning she treated it like a big joke, but I'd fallen for her. I pursued her as best I could, visiting her in Boston several times, but it was no use, and I let it go soon after that. I'd seen her once since those times, with her husband, but so much time had passed that I felt no great pang of jealousy or anything like that. By the time I saw her in Mexico last week the whole thing seemed so far gone that it might as well have happened to someone else.

Back in the truck Kayla went on. "I just never thought… I never thought this could happen to me. I never thought I could look at anyone after Dylan." She started to meekly sob into her hands.

"Oh Jesus Kay, come on, don't cry," I implored. "You'll be fine. Tomorrow night you'll be back in Nebraska, right? You didn't do anything."

"I know I didn't do anything, Nick," she blurted petulantly, "That's not the point." I tried to calm her down and succeeded after a while. We were both fools and had a good laugh at our dramatics before continuing into the video store and grabbing a couple of movies. Before walking back into the apartment she dried her eyes, smudging her make up in sad little streaks.

I opened the front door and was accosted by Lobo, sleepily shuffling around like a Mexican zombie. He made a menacing, rotting corpse face at us, symbolizing an expression of his tired and beaten body. Linda and Dan immediately seized this opportunity of consciousness and lit a fire under his ass to go out and drink on their last night in Austin. It was no surprise that within minutes he was showered and dressed and ready to go, go, go. I tried to hold onto my movie night, but Kayla wouldn't stay unless someone else did and Cassandra, the only other one weak enough in her convictions for a night out on the town, was committed to staying by her husband's side. "Listen Vittas," Lobo began negotiating, "just go to the first bar with us, then we'll drop you off and go to 'Nasty's' and shake our shit."

"I'm fucking beat," I protested.

"You'll be home by eleven, come on," they all said.

That first bar was actually pretty funny. It was the Saxon Pub on Lamar Blvd. There was a cool, eighteen year old ratty, white kid with a beat up guitar on stage with an equally cool, dreadlocked, Bob Marley looking drummer. The drummer was poised and hip about his business while the guitarist ripped on his guitar and screamed into the microphone with such all out intensity that the veins on his face and the arteries on his throat bulged out at the audience. He was actually pretty talented and even though his emo-acoustic rock wasn't up our alley, we were all drawn in and started to really cheer for him because of the insane energy he put into every chord and every angst ridden lyric. "I love him," Lobo flatly proclaimed. "He's just so cool. Look at him, look at him. I wanna put him in a box and take him home with me." When his set ended Lobo and this girl across the bar, which together comprised the kid's unofficial fan club, made uproarious, drunken demands for an encore. He obliged with a blush and then we left to drop me off.

Lobo pulled the truck around the apartment parking lot, I hopped out and to my surprise Kayla slid out too. "Kayla, what are you doing?" Lobo hollered from the driver's seat.

"I'm tired too, I think I'll just watch a movie too." He paused for a moment, calculating how much pressure to apply.

"What, you really don't want to come?" She shook her head. "Okay," he said as he maneuvered the truck for an exit."

"Good choice Kayla," I said. I set up my camping mat for her and a thin bed of blankets for myself in front of the TV. We started to chatter at first, pausing the movie for ten minutes to get a point across then continuing on only to pause it again several minutes later. It became clear that there was no point in trying to follow the plot and we let the movie run as we talked. We listened to each other intently and spoke honestly and directly from the naked truth of our souls and experiences before the flickering screen ahead of us. Nothing was guarded or needed to be. We purged ourselves of insecurities, of past relationships, of friendships gained and lost and the pain and frustration connected to dwindling health. We basked in reminiscence of the crutch that faith can be in your darkest hour. I told her the story of my misdiagnosis and the years of doctor's visits as things deteriorated and of the odd "coincidence" of stumbling onto a correct diagnosis a month after deciding to give faith a try because I had nothing to lose.

She started to talk about her life before Dylan. "My vice was never drugs or alcohol," she admitted, "It was sex. I've done a lot of things I'm not proud of. I've taken so many risks I never should have and let people use me and treat me like shit, but all that changed after I met Dylan." I guess every vice is used to stave off loneliness, hers just cut straight to the point. "I prayed and I prayed and I prayed to God to give me the strength not to act that way and to bring me a husband and make me a wife," she continued with a strain in her voice as she visited that time in her life. "A good wife. A wife a man would be proud to have. And then I met Dylan. We dated for two years and waited 'til we were married before we had sex." She was smiling and I realized something that I lost sight of in the coming days: there were external forces bringing those two together, there were desires for simplicity, stability, and straightforwardness within both of them, drawing them close to each other like a set of tectonic plates bound to move toward each other by forces within their structure and just outside them too. How foolish it was to feel any jealousy in the face of such things.

Lobo, Dan, Linda, and Cassandra barged in on us at 2:30 that night, loud belligerent and hungry. They drunkenly wolfed down slices of pizza and were snoring as Kayla and I said goodnight. I woke up at six to take a leak and when I lay back down I saw her staring at me across the floor. She reached her hand out and I grasped it. We were at it again, whispering endlessly with a joyous, secret enthusiasm as she caressed my fingers. She was slated to leave at five in the afternoon. Should I have done something, anything? I did nothing. We quit talking at nine.

By 9:30 everyone was up, waking me up along with them after three short, aggravated hours of sleep. The mad pace picked up right where it left off. There was no time for breakfast. We had to race to Alejandra's in San Antonio where an insurance agent would arrive at 11:00 to replace the shattered windshield. Quick goodbyes were said to Linda and Dan and they waved from the bus stop as we sped off. We continued the great race that started in Mexico four days ago and hadn't let up since. Kayla and I sat in the mini cab with a mound of pillows between us. I slipped my hand under the pillows and she immediately shot hers under too, grasping mine. I don't know why I did that. It was pointless and childish and cowardly. I guess I just wanted to pretend for a little longer.

We got there with minutes to spare. I was dog-tired and a hole grumbled in the cavernous hollow my stomach had turned into. I probably should have eaten some of the plain pasta Alejandra had sitting out on her stove, but it was so bland and a sit down, delicious restaurant meal was continuously dangled in front of me, promised to be right around the corner, right after this next, last chore. As I was carrying Kayla's bags out of the car my head began to feel lighter and lighter, as if it was floating away. A twisted noxiousness gripped my stomach. With shaky steps I made it back to the front door. My face felt flushed and pale at the same time and the corners of my vision started to creep in white. *Shit, I hope I haven't fucked myself*. I blacked out, collapsing at the foot of Alejandra's couch. The race was over. My body had tapped out. I'd driven on fumes the night before and now the tank was starkly empty.

When my eyes opened I saw that I was surrounded by a ring of Mexicans peering down at me. As I weakly made my way to the table Lobo bustled around me in a panic. "Do you need water, do you want some water, some milk, some pasta. Cassandra, heat up some Goddamn pasta for God's sake. No I'll heat it, you don't know how to heat it up fast enough. Pasta Nick, you must eat pasta. I should have given you something to eat. Damn it, this is all my fault." Cassandra, Kayla and Alejandra looked over me with concerned, motherly faces as Lobo paced around me like he was on a motorized track. It was all quite embarrassing. After eating a little pasta and drinking some water I went upstairs and crashed onto the bed like I was punishing it for leaving me. I drifted to sleep as bizarre chills shivered throughout my body. When I woke up they were all asleep in the living room. Kayla's flight left at five, we had to leave within the hour. I ate a sandwich someone left on the table and Kayla awoke, almost like she sensed me around. A misplaced, reminiscent sadness fell between us, as if we were ending some long relationship, but really it was just the end of a stupid, fleeting impulse that flickered and burned out under the weight of reality. Our melancholy murmurs stirred Lobo to life as he stretched and groaned from his spot on the floor. He immediately barraged me with a flurry of questions on how I was feeling and would have demanded lab tests if I could provide any. "Jesus you scared me," he sighed. "Your father was expecting me to take care of you and you die on my watch." For the rest of the day if I gave a hint of not being full he would drop what he was doing and practically cram food down my throat. "Not on my watch," he'd proclaim, "no one is dying on my watch. Now eat this."

We drove Kayla to the airport, said our goodbyes, and then were promptly informed that her flight was canceled due to mechanical difficulties. She was with us for one more night. We drove back to Lobo's apartment in Austin. Despite our best efforts Kayla and I aggravatingly found our familiar rhythm again and talked as Junior was given a bath. Everyone was in unanimous agreement that sleep, good sleep was in order. We set up a massive bed of blankets in front of the TV and watched a movie. Kayla and I were purposeful bookends to the group. Before dawn I woke up again to go to the bathroom. I was always waking up on account of all the water I had to drink with my medicine right before I hit the sack. Kayla was awake when I got back, just looking at me, and the endless whisper continued. Apparently this girl was trying to kill me by sheer exhaustion if not desire. All of the spontaneous exuberance of the previous night was replaced by a contemplative sadness. We were alone in the living room. Cassandra, Lobo, and Junior had relocated to their bedroom at some point in the night. Kayla stretched out on her blanket and the dawn shot through the blinds, painting pencil thin stripes of light on her soft, brown flesh as she stared over at me and I did nothing. We did nothing. From the moment we'd started talking it seems that we were destined for sadness; either because she'd given into temptation and reverted to her old ways or because I was too big of a coward to pounce upon an opportunity that had been laid out in front of me, and deal with the sordid aftermath when the time came. She would cry if we did. I would brood if we didn't. Such is life.

A year later I found myself faced with an oddly similar decision. I was in a relationship that I probably shouldn't have been in, and found myself on a trip without my significant other. I was with my cousins in Greece and one of my cousin's wife's friends was along for the trip. This girl was a model—the kind of girl that turns every head in a room and induces men to make fools of themselves in an attempt to grab her attention. In Greece no one has any respect for relationships and everyone, from aunts and uncles to cousins, was pressuring me to make a move on her. I did nothing for two reasons. One, I have no game whatsoever, and two, I didn't want to be a cheater. Every night everyone but me went out to the clubs and one night as they all returned this model crawled into my bed. She made her intentions clear by pulling the sheets over us and resting her head on my chest as her moist breath, perfumed with the taste of vodka and cigarettes, tickled my throat. I remembered how empty I'd felt after letting Kayla slip through my fingers, remembered how unsatisfying it was to do the 'right thing', so I did the 'wrong thing'. As soon as it was over I felt just as unsatisfied as I had a year earlier and I realized that sometimes life corners you into a situation where either path you choose will lead to equal dissatisfaction.

Dan and Linda had left on a bus up to Boston the day before—52 brutal hours of transfers and layovers. Now Kayla left for Nebraska. The group was shrinking by the day. We dropped her off at the Starbucks on the corner of Oltorf and I-35 and a friend of hers picked her up and drove her to the airport in San Antonio. It was sad to see her go. She went home to her husband and promptly had a baby. He was everything I wasn't because he wasn't mad like her family. My time in Texas was winding down too. My flight to DC was scheduled for the next day and we were all so tired from the manic run of energy it took to get from La Madrid to Austin that we just ended up eating a silent dinner and passing out in their bare apartment. The only excitement of the day came right after we dropped Kayla off for the final time.

Lobo wanted to take Junior to get his stitches removed. "Put your shoes on," he casually told his son as he grabbed his keys from the counter. Junior refused. "Azel," his voice grew louder, "put them on."

"Pfft," Junior replied. It was becoming his signature of defiance. An aristocratic, snobbish puff of air that flipped the hair off his forehead for a second, with a dismissive scowl painted on his baby face, like he couldn't believe the idiots fate had surrounded him with.

"Put them on," Lobo thundered. This move Junior had conjured up cut to the heart of all his frustration with his boy and tore open a heated rage in him.

"No," Junior screamed back.

"God Damn it, I said put them on now." Junior stubbornly looked away from the shoes as if the things were beneath him. He ignored further calls from his father to put them on until Lobo's eyes fell over the room in desperation and focused in on Dora the Dolly. And this is where the De Los Reyes gene displays its intricate and almost delicate savagery. A gene of twisted humor and conflict that breeds upon itself to create the most spectacular fireworks. "Put your shoes on or I'll throw your Dolly out," Lobo threatened, lunging for the doll and holding her by the throat.

"No," Junior wailed in anguish, but refused to move toward the doll or the shoes. The kid was no one's bitch and he wasn't going to be bullied into putting those shoes on. Lobo saw that this was going nowhere and turned up the pressure.

"Put your damn shoes on or I'll break her neck, I'll break your Dolly's neck," he growled as he stapled her plastic head to the floor with his knee and pulled her legs up with trembling fists.

"Nooo," Junior shrieked hysterically, crying and jumping in place, shaking his hands in agony, wailing and turning red in the face. But still, he refused those shoes like a hostage negotiator that knows one cannot surrender to terrorist action.

"I swear to God I'll break her neck," Lobo roared, a sly grin slipped from his face, which was so completely gripped by vengeful malice it looked demonic. He couldn't help but laugh at the ridiculousness of it all, if only for a fleeting second. Cassandra too didn't know what to feel. She was laughing and sobbing at the same time. I became so overwhelmed by the pressure cooker of emotion that seemed poised to blow the roof off the building that I ran up to the shoes and begged Junior to just put them on.

"Look, I'm putting my shoes on, look how easy it is."

You couldn't tell whether this was a comedy, (definitely dark), or a heart wrenching drama. It was both mixed up together into something unbearably intense. Lobo started to pull the legs with all his might and I could hear the first cracks of Dolly's neck giving way beneath the piercing screams of the boy. It was a madhouse—an epic showdown of wills with the head of a Dolly at stake. Cassandra convulsed in the corner, despondent tears streaming down her round cheeks and trickling into lines formed by her baffled smile. Lobo's horrid face shifted into a bemused smirk, as if even he couldn't believe the madness of the whole thing. I certainly couldn't and continued to beg Junior to put his shoes on and end the grisly affair. But Junior wailed and plowed dead ahead, seemingly willing to sacrifice his beloved Dolly in the name of freedom and a boy's right to choose when he puts his shoes on. Moments before Dora the Dolly would have been decapitated for good Junior relented and put those fucking shoes on. I felt like a dictator had just taken his finger off the button. Cassandra and I heaved grateful sighs in between befuddled laughter. What just happened?

And within seconds father and son embraced and sauntered out to the car as if Lobo had asked Junior to put his shoes on and he'd only done it after a stern look. They held hands and smiled at each other. As I watched them from inside the dark apartment doorway the sun beat down and bonded them together in the light. It was just the madness from their mad, bottled up souls that had to jump out and romp and rage, but fizzled away right after it was let out. There was an impermanence to these blowups, to the entire manic rollercoaster that the De Los Reyes clan perpetually rode up and down on. There was no getting off the ride for them, the ride was life and they experienced every moment to its core because there's no room for anything else. Nothing is sugar coated or dimmed down. Everything shines brightly with intensity: from idle nights watching movies, to belligerent bouts of drinking, to frantic flea markets, and incestuous love, and sweeping strokes across the highways of a forgotten land, and fights, and hugs, and laughter. It seems at the end there is always laughter. It's a wretched drama that melds back and forth between comedy and tragedy so often you lose sight of what's funny and what's harrowing. But in the end there is an unspoken recognition that everything is temporary, from elation to devastation, so why not spread it all out in the open and let time wash over the whole thing. I sat in the back seat of the Matrix as we drove to the clinic to get Junior's stitches removed and laughed silently as I recovered my senses. This was my last stop on the rollercoaster for a while. It had all been a blast. Now I'd go home and cut that

6,000-dollar check the insurance company gave me for the Honda and buy a new car. And who knows, if I got lucky maybe I could hop back on the rollercoaster for another spin sometime.

A Vessel of the Moment
July 2011

"Cut open doors and windows to create a room/ in its emptiness there is the function of a room/ Therefore, that which exists is used to create benefit/ that which is empty is used to create functionality"
—Lao Tzu

Sometimes I feel weak at night. Somehow in the darkness I forget everything I've learned over the last decade. A panic sweeps over me and my soul feels like it's got a plague of termites weaving through it, rotting me from the inside out. I lie in bed and weep as quietly as I can. During these nights I'm full of grief over the past and anxiousness over the future and there is little room for anything else. The latest symptom that has sprung back into my life, whether it's leg pain, backaches, migraines, or fatigue, overwhelms me and all I seem able to do is to wish for an easier life. I know that it is foolish to act this way, but somehow I lose all composure in the night and I can't find my way out of the darkness.

I had a night just like this a week before I was slated to leave for a trip up to Massachusetts. I'd been living in Austin three years, and now mostly pointed myself north and east when getting ready to hit the road. On this particular night a stabbing pain in my left shoulder startled me out of a deep sleep. I tried to gain a hold on the situation by focusing on my breath, but the pain was too intense or my will too weak, and I found myself wishing as I wept in the darkness. I prayed for God to take the pain away, and then I prayed for the day that I'd be dead and gone instead. Through the pain and the tears I pictured my funeral. Who would be there? What would they say to each other? What would they think of me? Somehow that was all I could think about.

A week went by and I was still rattled by this night. Doubts and worries lingered around me as I packed the Honda. What if the pain came back that strong again? What if I could no longer handle the pain like I had in the past? What if these trips were the latest thing that the disease forced me to give up? The drive to Massachusetts was long and hard. On the first day I drove through blinding headaches until I couldn't stand it anymore. I stopped at a rest station somewhere in Arkansas and slept in the driver's seat for two hours, which gave me just enough strength to finish the day's driving.

When the headaches came back the next day I focused on my breath, found that judgeless state and kept rolling north. In the afternoon of the third day I was approaching Johnny's house in Belchertown, Massachusetts. Johnny had lived with me and Lobo in that mad house where couches were burned every weekend and kegs hung in the trees like ripe fruit. That house, which I'd left in 1998, was actually only five minutes from Johnny's place. He was married to his college sweetheart, had two kids, and had chosen the same profession we all seemed to fall into, teaching.

The headaches came back hard again as I raced north up I-91, pulsating from the back of my skull and clawing out onto the side of my face. I went back to my breath and suddenly the words, "I am a vessel of the moment" popped into my head. I'm not sure where they came from, but they were incredibly comforting and inspirational. I repeated them over and over like a mantra as I drove. "I am a vessel of the moment". To be a vessel of the moment I had to empty myself of everything else. I had to purge myself of all judgments, all desires, of all the grief that came along with being sick and make room for the present moment to reside within me and guide me as well.

When I got to Johnny's house I was exhausted. Light from the kitchen windows hit me like a brick in the face. I wanted to sit down and catch up with him and his wife, Agnes, but I couldn't. I went straight to his guest room and slept for a solid hour. There was a band up from Austin playing in the next town over, Northhampton. We'd been planning on going. When I woke up I felt a little better and we decided to give it a shot.

Johnny and Agnes sat up front as we drove to Northhampton. This was the first time they'd been out as a couple since the birth of their second child six months ago. They were excited, like a couple of teenagers sneaking out. I felt weak and my head throbbed. I repeated my mantra from the drive up to myself silently and a great joy swept up through me. I was a vessel for the moment. If I dumped out all the worry and concern about the pain I could make room for the present. I began to feel elated with the present, and actively let the laughter flow through me. I made room for laughter like you dig a trench for a waterway, and it trickled out of me in the same way. Johnny sat up front cracking jokes and each one hit me like I was on laughing gas. The pain didn't exactly diminish, but it didn't consume me either. I could have been concerned with how I would last at a two or three hour show, how my head would hold up with all the amplified noise, would my neck start hurting worse, but I could not think of those things since I had carved myself into a vessel of the moment, and I was empty of everything aside for the present.

I began to feel a light form of giddiness, as if I were made of air and could float along in my own existence. We parked the car and Agnes and I ran to a chocolate shop while Johnny went to buy the tickets. I smiled out at the world and greeted each person I came across with genuine wonder and interest. I did not glaze over my interactions, but instead innocently examined every detail, and all the details added up to produce a wonderful mosaic. The cashier smiled back at me and I felt the genuine pleasure of receiving a smile from a stranger. I felt it because I had emptied myself of all other thoughts and concerns and there was room to feel it. What a powerful thing a smile from a stranger can be.

Inside the small venue the music throbbed against my head. We sat near the back, on a ring of stools surrounding a small table. There was no backrest. The muscles in my shoulders bunched up and started to ache. The music beat against my head as well. But it was good music. I liked it. It moved me. I let go of the heartache that came along with being in pain and made room for the music to fill me with as much joy as it could. Of course I would have enjoyed the show more if I wasn't in pain, but I would have barely noticed the music if I was consumed by the hurt. I gave the music space to swim inside of me, and so it swam and filled me with a humble gratitude for its beauty. Johnny and Agnes got drunk. They beamed out at the world like a pair of teenagers in love and the three of us sat in the corner, a little bundle of lanterns shining throughout the whole show.

It's not always this easy. Many times since this night I've tried to find the sublime rhythm I stumbled upon in Massachusetts and have had mixed results. Sometimes I find it and sometimes I find a cheap substitute. But there is no doubt in my mind that when I do carve myself into a vessel of the moment I can function, both physically and spiritually, much better with a body that is often in pain.

Questions
November 2010

Chronic Lyme disease continually encourages me to question myself, from my beliefs, to my desires, to who I am. Aside from producing aggravating and painful symptoms that force me to take a step back and analyze whether a certain life view can bring me happiness within the confines of the disease, Chronic Lyme has also somewhat isolated me and given me plenty of time to introspectively look at my life. When people my age were at the bars drowning their thoughts in beer I was often sitting in my room dissecting a philosophy to see where it stood within the context of chronic pain.

Part of taking an introspective look at my life has always included asking myself questions without clear answers. Sometimes I'll ponder these questions, running them over in my mind until an answer materializes, but more often I delve into books from men and women who are far wiser than myself for a little guidance. The disease has made me into quite a reader, which is another one of those silver lined blessings; I may have more time to read, and more reason to scrutinize my beliefs because my body is often in pain, but I've learned a lot about myself and life in the process.

Chronic pain is always the biggest motivator of my deepest questions. Somehow it always comes back to this specific form of suffering for me. I can chart the evolution of how I mentally deal with and view chronic pain starting from the gut wrenching fear of, and utter aversion to, persistent pain in the late 1990s, to my experiment in faith and subsequent reliance on it through the mid 2000s, all the way to my latest progression of firmly planting myself in the present moment and objectively observing the pain the same way I observe all the sensations streaming through my consciousness. All these outlooks came after scrutinizing my belief system when it came to pain and how I dealt with it. I asked myself questions and I looked for answers. This latest strategy of immersing myself in the present offers me a considerable amount of peace when the hurt is bad, particularly because I've come upon it after three years of deteriorating symptoms that faith doesn't seem to be curtailing, or more importantly, helping me deal with.

That being said, there is still something about the whole *immerse myself in the present moment when the pain hits me* that doesn't sit right with me. Instinctively I want to try to do something about the pain, even if it is as simple as projecting a positive belief into the universe that I will be healthy. But, this attempt to impose my will upon reality doesn't quite sit well with me either. I've been reading a lot of eastern philosophy lately and much of what Taoist and Buddhist masters have to say resonates with me deeply. My suffering, they insist, is not a consequence of the physical discomfort that the disease creates in my body, but my mind's reaction to these unpleasant sensations, specifically the desire to be rid of them. According to many of the mystics, desire is the root of all suffering. The particular events of our lives are irrelevant, it's the desire to change our reality, the desire to change *what is* that causes us to suffer. This theory makes sense to me, it is very practical, but for some reason I can't fully embrace it.

Is abandoning all desires the only way to liberate myself from suffering? Is the deeply ingrained instinct to want to try, to want to find some way of aiding my body to heal itself, and therefore assert my will upon reality, an indication that I am still heavily identifying with my ego, and so missing the point that my individual self is an illusion? By refusing to give up on the possibility of having a healthy body am I insuring that I stay glued to the wheel of suffering? Is the chronic pain trying to teach me to let go of my desires and find peace within the moment? If so, why doesn't it sit completely right with me? Why do I feel as if I'm missing one piece of the puzzle? All these questions irk me, like an itch that can't be scratched. When part of my body flares up in pain I don't exactly know how to receive the sensation. Do I humbly and totally accept *what is*, leaving all desire to change the circumstance of illness into health? Do I stubbornly continue to strive to change that circumstance into health? These questions are vitally important to how I react to the most challenging aspect of my life, but I don't have any answers, so I let them float in my mind and hope that given time and space they will rearrange themselves into some semblance of answers.

When the car had been stolen out in Oakland, all of Costa's trademark confidence had gone with it. He felt responsible, and the guilt made him trigger shy to comical proportions, where he'd look at me, bewildered, and ask for assistance deciding upon the most mundane choices, like what burger joint to eat at or which radio station to choose. Often his indecision only served to muddle things further for us. While stranded we'd watched the movie *The Big Lebowski*. The main character, The Dude, has his car stolen while saddled with a screw up sidekick, Walter Sobchak, who manages to complicate The Dude's life with one well intentioned fuck up after another. I'd gone to calling Costa, "Walter Demas," because he'd dragged me to Oakland and completely marred our trip. The Walter stigma had even seeped into Costa's usually unshakable game with the ladies. Passing through Crescent City he had become enamored with a checkout girl and approached her, only to get flustered at the crucial moment. He stammered an awkward introduction, then walked away in defeat. In the end we made the best of it, drove in a rental the insurance company provided, up through Northern California, into Oregon, then back to the Bay area, where I flew to Austin and Costa flew home.

After a little more than a month with the De Los Reyes clan I came home and immediately got some stunning news: the Honda had been found out in California. I started making arrangements to go save her from the auction blocks out west right away. All I needed now was a running mate.

I spent the majority of the next week in Costa's apartment crashing on his couch. Costa was unemployed. The company he worked for had folded weeks after he returned from Oakland and he was now engrossed in a vigorous job hunt. He had a big interview on the 28th of August and I gradually wore him down until he agreed that if he landed the job he'd ask to start in two weeks and fly out west with me. "No job, no money, no trip with Niko," Costa told me, so the caveat was landing him a job. During this time we just loafed around the apartment and the neighborhood bars and coffee houses, and the week dragged by slowly.

Finally the day of the interview arrived. Costa woke me in the living room as he prepared for the big interview he was banking on for gainful employment, and more importantly, the one I was banking on to catch a partner to drag across the country. A trip to California, up to through the great northwest, with a quick hello to Vancouver and back across the entire width of the continent was probably the furthest thing from Costa's mind that morning. He was a pacing, bundle of nail biting nerves. "I wish I could do this right now," he anxiously grumbled, "I've got so much riding on this, Niko. I need this." His round eyes darted around the room. His lips were pursed as he nervously ran his fingers through his dark hair. I nodded to everything he said. "I need this Niko." His mind was just running around the same track, spitting out the same comments at all the scheduled stops.

We were at my parent's house the next day, eating a late lunch at four o'clock, four hours past the 24 hour deadline the director had given herself to hire someone and Costa took this as a catastrophic sign. "I didn't get it, man. I know I didn't get it. She would have called by now if I had gotten it. I got a bad feeling, Niko." His stocky frame slouched dejectedly in his chair. He hadn't stopped fretting about the interview for the last two days, and was now boring my parents with every detail, though they seemed genuinely interested. I would go alone if he was right, but how much better it would be with a running mate.

With a mouthful of pasta in his face, Costa's phone rang. The number on the caller ID nearly made his eyes pop out of his round head as he swallowed the pasta in one panicked gulp and scurried out of the kitchen to answer the phone. I could hear Costa's hushed business tones from the living room and they sounded grateful. Any doubt was squashed when he cried, "Yeah" as he ran back into the kitchen. "I got the job." We all congratulated him. "I start September 17th." My ears perked up to this little tidbit of information. I let him revel in his success for a little while before pressing more immediate matters.

"Look, that's great about your job, but it's time to talk about this trip, you're coming, right?" I asked.

"Yeah," he muttered with a wonderstruck smile. Everything was piecing together fabulously. We were both dumbfounded by how smoothly it was all falling into our laps.

Two days later we were in Fremont, California. While we waited at the dealership for the finishing touches to be put on the Honda, Costa called Mitch, this guy we'd gone to high school with that I hadn't seen in almost a decade. Mitch lived in Portland, and even though I'm well aware of Costa's penchant for keeping in touch, I was taken by surprise when Costa demanded, more seriously than not, that Mitch let us stay at his place despite the fact the he would be out of town for the weekend. Apparently I was the holding point. The last time Mitch saw me I was a rowdy, drunken mess, perpetually high on something, and Mitch was leery of letting a walking catastrophe into his apartment. "He hasn't had a drink in years, he's harmless, Mitch," Costa pleaded. Mitch agreed to leave the keys to his apartment in the third vase down the hall from the elevator and we had our first destination.

There were some hold ups with the car, but we got an early enough start the next day. Costa got a phone call from Suzy, a girl he had a little thing with back in the day. She lived in Portland and had heard that he was on his way. "I've always wanted to close that deal but never got it done," Costa confessed after hanging up, licking his chops in a ravenously hungry way. There were few moments that he wasn't hungry for women, and somehow they always ended up hungry for him too. "A couple of years ago she visited DC with her boyfriend. I met them at some bar and she was all pressed up against me by the bathroom while her boyfriend was upstairs," Costa said, pondering possibilities. Apparently the boyfriend was recently out of the picture.

We clipped past the canopy of tunnels the Redwoods create, past the spot where we dropped off Powerful, Puffer Fish Ron, past Eureka, and Crescent City, pushing hard for the Oregon line. I drove us to the Smith River, where we took a quick dip in the icy, emerald waters and then plowed ahead. By eight, I sat in the passenger seat with an invigorating shiver rattling through me, the generous gift of a swim in the Smith, as Costa pushed the Honda north up 101, then over to I-5. Regrettably we drove all of Oregon in the dark. I reclined the chair all the way back and gazed at the stars gliding by through the open sunroof. Later I could see the silhouetted mountains in the rising moonlight and wondered what wonderful details I was missing. In the name of time and mileage we had to tear ahead. I was both sad and excited. We had been at it from the break of dawn for the second straight day and I'd reached my limit. Costa slammed down one caffeinated drink after another in an attempt to get to Portland that night. I gave up trying to support his heroic efforts and passed out, grabbing two surprisingly sweet hours of deep sleep as we approached the first city of the great northwest.

We had first expected to stay in a motel, then upgraded to digging for keys in hallway vases for our own private apartment, and now were greeted by a handsomely voluptuous blonde with perplexingly dark eyebrows and crisp, blue eyes. She had a thick, husky voice, and was drunk, full of laughs and hugs. "Hey Suzy, how you doin' darlin'," Costa smoothly greeted her. His dimpled grin tickled her. I sat hunched over on the front steps of Mitch's downtown apartment with all our bags stacked at my feet as Costa parked the car across the street. Suzy plopped down next to me, unleashing a drunken, wafting sigh with the effort. I hadn't seen her in more than a decade, and catching up can be a hard thing to do when there's just so much, but we managed. Costa labored out of the car and I screamed at him to put "the club" on the wheel. "This is Portland, not Oakland," Suzy scoffed at me. God, how awful it would have been to get the car back only to have it stolen again.

"Suzy, we don't fuck around anymore," I told her, joking, but with a hint of seriousness too, "we take car theft very seriously." Giggling, she led the way up to Mitch's apartment.

Mitch had a nice two-bedroom spread with wood floors and a balcony. He was down in Frisco for the weekend, and it's too bad too. It would have been nice to see him and see what he loved about the city. Costa insidiously disappeared to the bathroom and I took an immediate liking to Suzy when she came right out during our introductory, bullshit formalities, almost in a confession, and said, "I'm twenty-seven and I really don't know what I want to do. Just finished culinary school, so I think I'll give that a try."

"Shit, who are you talking to? I'm almost thirty and still live in my parent's basement." I'm always more comfortable, at least initially, with people that didn't feel the need to propel themselves into a career during their twenties, but rather stumbled around from job to job.

Costa crept out of the bathroom and sidled up next to Suzy. The three of us talked until the momentary jolt of energy I got from the new city and the new apartment died down and I dragged myself to sleep. Suzy was a cool girl. There was something cozy and nonchalant about her, as if she'd seen enough to be unfazed, but not too much to jade her enthusiasm. A little tinge of jealousy burnt in me as I went to sleep, but what did it matter, she was Costa's girl for the night and we'd be gone tomorrow anyhow. Besides, everyone has a role to play, mine has rarely been upfront and confident. I fully expected to hear stories of her conquest the next morning, but was surprised to find out that she had cut him off at the lips and he'd called it quits when it became obvious that the night would not progress past a heavy make out session.

We said our quick goodbyes to Suzy and kept moving down the line. On the first day we'd thrown the Honda in the fire and she'd responded marvelously. Aside from a little unexplained fishtailing, the freshly retrieved car had rattled off 14 hours and over 700 miles like the seasoned champion she'd always been.

We drove around the Portland morning aimlessly as was our custom whenever in a new city, a sort of tour by destiny that we gave ourselves with random turns whenever the impulse moved us. "Portland is like a mixture between Baltimore and San Francisco," Costa daftly observed. He was right. The city had that warehouse, harbor town infrastructure that defined Baltimore, but with a bohemian flare to it. Bookstores, CD shops, coffee houses, and bars seemed to crawl out of the blue collar skeleton the city held on to. After enough wandering we stopped and asked directions to I-5.

Balling fast up I-5 we made Seattle in no time. Costa drove as I sat shotgun. The blessed sense of peace that sweeps over me whenever I'm in a car, taking it easy, with no real agenda, but at the same time hauling ass to something or somewhere, worked its magic and I eased back into the seat in a trance. I caught a glimpse of myself in the side mirror. The face staring back at me looked old. And the eyes shot back like a stranger's, and I had the eerie sense that I was watching everything from outside myself. I might have stared at that stupid mirror all the way to Seattle if Costa hadn't turned the radio on.

The Rolling Stones snapped me back. "Ahh, yes. That's my jam," I yelled, pounding the dashboard as I took notice of my surroundings again, barely able to contain the exuberance that bubbled inside of me and spilled out into an eager, little grin that fit so finely on my boney face.

"It's good to see you happy like this," Costa said with a chuckle. "You love this shit, huh?"

"Oh, I love it." I was drunk with the whole thing, drunk with anticipation for what lay over the horizon.

"This must be, like, the ultimate freedom, compared to when you were sick and locked away in your home, huh?" Costa asked in a thoughtful tone.

"Holy shit," I murmured, "you're right." How was this obvious fact dawning on me just now? In his own, simple way Costa had read my subconscious motivations like a book. I loved him for it. "I'm like one of those Greeks that lived through the food shortages of World War II, and now has to shove every morsel of food down his throat, and the throats of his friends and family. I guess once you go through a shortage you can never have enough," I laughed.

We were only in Seattle for a couple of hours, and so we cut straight for Pike Place market because I'd heard of it. We walked through the charming streets of the emerald city, and then along the pier, stopping to watch all the ferries bustling out into the foggy Pacific. The air was filled with the appetizing scents of seafood. We put our names on the waiting list of the restaurant that had the most patrons and sat at the bar to wait for a table. "And let's welcome our new guests," said this young, black kid sitting next to the open seats intended for us. He was neatly dressed in grey wool pants, a button down shirt, and a derby hat. There was a buxom brunette to his right, whom I thought was giving me and Costa the eyes, but then realized that her eyes were always lustily peering at anything that moved—it was just her way.

"Hello to our new hosts," I shot back with a grin.

"Ya'll gotta try these crabs," he said as she smiled over his shoulder. His name was Steven and hers was Rachel, and the four of us hit it off marvelously.

"You guys aren't from here are you?" Steven said more than asked with a half smile slyly crinkled on his face. No, we clearly weren't, and Costa jumped at the chance to tell our story, and how we found ourselves out west again. He was very proud of our circumstances. And in his element, in an urban landscape of restaurants and bars, Costa really is a master socializer, able to fluidly talk with anyone. He has an almost sixth sense of what to ask or say to make people open up just enough so they're feeling sociable, but not so much that they feel vulnerable. There never seems to be an awkward moment with Costa around. And with the ice so casually broken, the four of us melted it all away. We melded into a foursome, swapping stories across the bar as a gregarious spirit intertwined us with the thread made from the common and easy bond all humans should share. Rachel and Steven worked together at the Hilton. I never could get a read on whether they were friends or something more, and finally settled on the notion that Steven was pushing for more, and Rachel was intrigued, but indecisive. "You guys were our best guests," Steven complimented us when we finished up, giving the impression that the two of them had been there all day, welcoming one set of patrons after another.

We left Seattle and continued north to Vancouver. The pavement hummed in harmony with the Honda. The evergreen vastness blurred by as mountains shot up and down. Costa sat with his cell phone loosely to his ear. He was chatting proficiently about nothing in particular with Candie, a friend of his sister's whom he hadn't seen in years. Candie lived in Vancouver, and even though Costa failed to secure us a place to stay that night, Candie agreed to meet up with us and show us the city.

It wasn't long before we found ourselves on Granville Street. It was a wild street, where rowdy Americans, most under the age of 21, came to trample and yell. I was accosted by a group of these kids right on the steps of our hotel. They were laughing and yelling in belligerent anticipation of all the excesses they were poised to enjoy. A girl from the group ran up and asked me to take a picture of the group in front of the hotel; apparently the Days Inn was an incredible landmark that had to be remembered. I laughed and did as I was told. They were just a bunch of dumb kids, but I liked the zeal that carried them on wings down the street. I watched them float away and felt old and tired.

We were awaiting Candie, Costa's sister's friend. She lived several blocks away. It seemed Costa had someone he knew in every city. Candie had a slender body, dressed on the stylish side, with designer jeans and a snug leather jacket, and had a face somewhat reminiscent of a goldfish. She also had the mismatching qualities of a valley girl's speech and facial expressions paired with an incredibly sharp wit. She rolled her eyes constantly and interjected the word "like," several times into every sentence. "I mean it's, like, so hard to meet guys out here. It's like, whatever, just come up to me and, like, talk to me instead of just sitting across the bar and just, like, staring at me the whole night. Gawd," she moaned when Costa asked her if she was seeing anyone. "It's like, Gawd, enough with the spooky white boys, please." Hearing her carry on like this you might make the mistake that she was a boring airhead, but she was actually quite smart, and had a sarcastic wit that she constantly jabbed at the both of us, at co-workers that weren't around to defend themselves, and with most vehement rancor toward Vancouver tourists, whom she viewed as a species of sub-human nitwits.

We walked through the brisk, Vancouver night, toward a bar she was fond of. "And this is the steam clock of Vancouver, it's, like, famous," she said as we passed it. "There's always tourists taking pictures of it, and I'm, like, why would you take a picture of a clock?" she continued, almost rolling her eyes clear out of her head. "It's the most photographed thing in Vancouver. Sometimes I like to run up to them and say, 'is that the steam clock?'" She said this last part with an exaggerated gasp, throwing her hands over her heart as her goldfish eyes bulged in mockery. "And they're like, 'yeah, do you want us to take your picture in front of it,' and I'm like, 'yeah, but I forgot my camera. Could you take it with yours and email me a copy?' Of course they say yes, then I give them a phony email." She shamed me from taking my picture of it.

Candie led us off the manic, neon turbulence of Granville Street and through a maze of haunting side streets. Seedy characters with weather beaten faces, and hard, nasty years beaten into their dirty wrinkles, stared out at us from the shadows of grimy side alleys and the dark steps of neglected buildings. There was a garbage strike. Black bags of trash were stacked on the pavement and at the entrance to these alleys, almost like sandbag barricades. Around one more corner and we found a quiet row of bars.

I was tired. I had a hard time keeping my eyes open. This trip had come on the tail end of one of my stronger summers, but there were still limitations that my body and the disease placed on me. Costa and Candie didn't seem to notice. They chatted along until the bar stopped serving and it was time to find a new spot. Mercifully they agreed to stand off their threat of holding me hostage for the night and instead split a cab ride back to the hotel with me. I stumbled upstairs and fell asleep in my clothes as they continued their night on the town.

The TV was blaring when the morning light cut through the drapes and splashed upon my face. I was fully dressed on top of the sheets and it was aggravatingly early. Costa was nowhere to be seen. I lay down, but sleep wouldn't come. I guess I was just anxious to get on with it. We'd established such a wonderfully satisfying rhythm to our travels that my bones ached to pick up and keep going. My flesh was fidgety and restless, and despite wholehearted pleas with myself for a delicious doze, I just lay there, a tired fool refusing sleep. A couple of hours later Costa dragged himself into the room like a two-day-old newspaper being blown down the gutter. He was gaunt, with bloodshot eyes that rested above a real shit eating grin. Even though his words came out soft and exhausted, there was a strut to them. "I worked it out with Candie last night," he whispered, radiating a boastfulness that only a true womanizer can be blessed with. He proceeded to fill me in on all the details of his late night escapades. Apparently Candie was the Honda's gift for Costa's loyalty. He killed Walter that night, once and for all. All signs of the hesitant, second-guessing machine that Oakland had created vanished. Walter had been executed, buried deep in Candie's rosebush during the dark hours of the Vancouver night.

The Tiniest of Buddhas
July 2009

There is a tiny Buddha that lives inside my chest and loves to listen to the blues. He dances and sways to the rhythm and sets me rolling like a wave when he moves inside of me, no matter how tired I was before the radio was turned on. His little rocking chair oscillations keep me driving late into the night as Jack and I slowly labor north into Wisconsin in the beat up old RV that I've been driving from Austin at a steady 55 miles per hour for the past four days. Tomorrow we should be creeping into Montana.

There is an invisible Sage lounging in my breast like there's a sofa in my heart. He feasts upon the North Dakota prairies that stretch wide and flat as far as my eyes can see. He marvels at the blooming, cotton ball clouds and their rolling, layered underbellies, which are almost as flat as the land they hover above. There is a tiny Saint inside me that registers pain, but never feels it. He observes everything and grasps at nothing. His tiny spirit is cleansed by suffering, and he welcomes the hurt the same way he welcomes everything, with arms as open as the sun.

All Jack can talk about is the sick burn he's gonna put on Costa for not coming on the trip this summer. He started taking pictures, even though he's always hated to. "I've got bigger fish to fry than my own happiness. I've got to get a sick burn on Costa," says Jack of his sudden interest in photography. "I want to come home and show him these pictures and see the sadness in his eyes, and I'll know he's defeated. He won't say it, but we'll both know." Only Jack would go on a road trip with a competitive vendetta high on his list of things to be attained. "Wait 'til we get to Montana. I can't wait to take some pictures."

There is a tiny Buddha in me who takes it all in, Jack's nonsense talk, the birds gracefully darting across the highway, the strenuous grumble of the motor, the throbbing pulse running over my skull, the clambering jingle of pots and pans from the sink in the rear—all of it received with infinite, celestial, gratitude, like a retired conductor reclining in the back row of the symphony. He knows the whole plain is his body, and he knows that each second is spontaneously reborn. He never leaves a trace of where he's been or a clue of where he's going. Sometimes I feel him in my gut, but mostly he is sitting in my chest, glowing like a radiator in the dark. He sits for no other reason than to sit and is never pressed for anything. He is my hero and my inspiration. When I focus on him and how he pays attention to the world, I get happy. I want to emulate him in every way, though I rarely succeed.

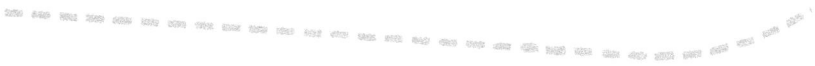

The Compromise
December 2010

"Therefore the sage avoids extremes, excesses, and complacency."
—Lao Tzu

*T*hrough asking myself what I could learn from the pain I stumbled onto the fact that when in pain I found myself in an almost mindless state, completely immersed in the present. Once I saw this piece of wisdom that the experience of pain offered me I connected to it deeply, and tried to incorporate the concept of staying in the moment into my life beyond the times when I ached. The peace that flowered from this mindset was real and directly connected to a level of happiness that I only experienced when completely engrossed in some creative task, be it writing, playing music, painting with a child, playing basketball, whatever. Quieting the mind seemed to offer some bridge into the creative state, where one could feel the peace and immersion of being lost in a creative art, but feel it during the everyday humdrum motions that occupy most of the day. In this way life could become art.

But did the release of the future and the past mean that I had to abandon my goal of being healthy as well? Did living in the moment demand that I passively accept all conditions that life placed on me and give up my will to shape these conditions? Was there no way to blend immersion in the present with faith that I would be healthy again?

I thought about it for some time before I came to a compromise. Perhaps I could balance the faith that had sprouted during my two-month experiment ten years ago with this new vision centered around focusing in on the moment. It seems to me that the two agents that prevent this balance from taking place are a preoccupation with time and frustration with a lack of results. Maybe I can tell myself that I will be healthy when I'm hurting without ripping myself away from the present moment if I observe the thought "I will be healthy" the same way I observe everything else in the present; neutrally, without any great attachment to results or aversion to outcomes.

For example if I'm washing dishes and the back of my head lights up in pain as if a massive brain freeze were doing laps in there, I can think to myself, "I will be free of this pain one day," as I watch the soap bubbles dance in the sink, listen to the water trickle from the faucet, feel my breath rise in and out of my chest, and feel the pain throb in my head. All the years that have gone by without great progress, without leaving this disease once and for all, don't affect me because I am truly immersed in the present. This present moment happens to be filled with a headache, soap bubbles, trickling water, my breath, and the thought that I will be healthy again. I observe the thought just as I observe these other sensations. Staving off frustration equals accepting all that is right now, but accepting all that is right now does not have to mean a passive acceptance of a condition as unchangeable. I can release the energy of positive thought and faith into the universe to change my current situation and stay in the present if I observe the will to improve my health the way I observe everything else, as part of the present. Your will can abide in the present just like everything else, as long as it doesn't become attached to results, and as long as it doesn't fall prey to frustration. Frustration is the obsession with time, but there is no time. There is only now.

Chicago Blue
September 8–9, 2007

"I love the blues because it tells the truth."
—Precious Bryant

By the time Costa and I saw the skyscrapers of the windy city, we had amassed some 3,800 miles on the freshly retrieved Honda, and still had 700 to go. All I could think was sweet home Chicago. The towers grew fast as we approached the blues Mecca and I was filled with a bubbling anticipation as I hoped to experience all the stories of mad blues shows I'd heard from friends who'd made the pilgrimage. The only name I could remember was the Kingston Mines, so we headed out that way.

I've been told by people who grew up in Chicago that the Kingston Mines, great as it can be, should only be the beginning of your blues experience in the windy city because it can be diluted by tourists who can affect the playing and set list of the bands. If this is true then I absolutely ache to see the journey of Chicago blues bands all the way to its holy end, because the Kingston Mines was nothing short of heaven that night.

They play blues every night, from eight to four, except on Saturdays when they go till five in the morning. And real blues too, the face scrunching, soul churning, foot stomping, genuine article. The joint's nothing more than two long, dark, wooden rooms, separated by a thin divide, each with a small stage and dance floor up front. There are two bands and each stays on their respective stage, trading off hour sets as the crowd rushes back and forth between the rooms. One band plays for an hour then breaks for an hour while the neighboring band takes over. The musicians are all local Chicago bluesmen, some of whom have been playing there for over thirty years, and all of whom played with the most sincere passion, crafted skill and joyous, reckless freedom that set my soul on fire.

It was the rawest sound I'd ever heard, and I was instantly captivated and electrified. My eyes bulged and my ears strained, but it was effortless because I was lifted by this consuming desire to grasp it all. There was a red glow about the place, as if what little light there was available was tinted by the music. The dark wooden walls sweat soul and reverberated with decades of pure, wonderfully intense emotion pounded into them. This was the blues, the history of it and the life of it. I foamed at the mouth to take it all in.

When I first got into the place I didn't even realize there were two stages, I just walked toward the music, sat down and knew I was exactly where I wanted to be. Three middle aged black men stood on a small stage, with a younger, baldheaded brother tucked away behind the drum set. In the center was a burly, light skinned bassist dressed all in white. He had a thick beard and swayed deeply to the driving groove he slapped on his bass while wailing into the microphone. He grinned broadly in between lyrics, beaming at his band mates like a child and they beamed right back, except for the drummer who was all business, but even he too shot an occasional smile that betrayed how happy he was to be playing the music.

The lead guitarist was a short man with a goofy, gold and purple Hawaiian shirt. His face contorted into all sorts of shapes as his guitar sang the praises of his heart. And the pianist was the funniest of them all--tiny and dark as a man can be, with round, little spectacles and a bow tie. He looked like a Southern-Baptist preacher. During his group's last set, he took his keyboard off its stand and started walking around the room, playing it on his head or behind his back. Then he laid it on the lap of a girl he dragged up on stage, a gorgeous, well-dressed blonde thing. She blushed a little as he sang, "let me love you baby," fixing an unfaltering gaze, filled with lust and appetite, right on her throughout the song. Then she turned cherry red and her blue eyes darted all over the room as he proclaimed, "Please let me love you baby...just let me show you how I'ma gonna do it." The preacher knelt down, with the keyboard on her lap, and started playing it with his tongue, directly over her crotch. Her boyfriend brooded in the shadows. The little keyboard preacher chuckled at him after the song was over, "I just got her started, you gotta finish her off." The crowd roared. He was the filthiest, maddest preacher I'd ever seen.

"Isn't this amazing," I yelled over to Costa who was planted right next to me, fixated on the stage like I was. There was a ruckus air about the place, the crowd was into it, they cared. When an audience is unabsorbed by the music they suck the life out of the room. Adversely, when they care and focus and are moved, they spur the band to greater, intensified heights. Everyone in the crowd may not have been crazy about the blues, but they knew a good show when they saw one, and devoted part of themselves to the performers. This vibe, this devotion grew steadily stronger as the night progressed until toward the end of the night, the mob appreciation had grown so tenaciously gripping that newcomers either jumped right in or immediately turned away. The bands felt this too. The sets grew wilder and more intense until the final one blew me straight to the moon.

"Sometimes I get the blues so bad I wana drink some gas-o-leen. But my mamma raised me to be such a good boy," the burly bassist hollered, "I'ma let ya'll have it instead." The crowd roared its approval and Costa was one of the many to take a drink in salute. They played one more song, in which the keyboard preacher took his keyboard off its stand and paraded around the room, twirling it around his back and upon his palm, never losing the rhythm of the song. And then, before they had even finished their set, the word spread through the room that the other band was about to start and in a mad scramble, the entire crowd pushed and shuffled and frantically herded through a slim door to the other stage.

There sat an old black man hunched over his guitar. He looked like a share-cropper from the old South. He had short, white hair and wore a tired, sullen expression as he tinkered with the strings of his axe. The band kicked in a slow, steady blues and he nodded his heavy old head in approval and began the weary process the elderly have of standing up. The fountain of youth can be nothing more than a song, I thought, as I saw this silver headed patriarch of the blues dust the creakiness off his bones and stand alive and strong before us. He sang in a furious, yet controlled manner, and shuffled in tiny circles around his mic, handling his guitar loosely, yet playing the passionate solos of the wise and unhurried sage who still holds the ember smoking in his chest.

Everyone cheered madly for him. It was marvelous to see someone well into their seventies still getting it done with truth and rawness that bit and howled, and told so forcefully the epic power that our emotions possess. "He looks and even sounds so much like R.L Burnside," I told Costa, "I'll show you when we get home."

"That's my black papou (Greek for grandfather)," Costa beamed, "I love that guy."

I closed my eyes and stomped my foot, it seemed to move of its own accord. The music dripped through me, pulsating, moving something inside of me. It either speaks to your soul or it doesn't. You're either lifted to the top floor or you don't get onto the elevator. It not only speaks to my soul, but calls out to me, intimately whispering to me with its lips pressed tightly against the ears of my heart and I can hear nothing else, and the world stops. And this is the power of the blues, trusted messenger of the super emotion, that sacred feeling of laughter wrapped in tears and all in between, the full human spectrum. When I hear this sound, I'm catapulted into this state where I feel it all at once, this frothing, blazing mass of emotions that seems almost too big to be contained, as if all I'm feeling is being pushed through a too small hole, too fast and my chest swells. My head nodded to the rhythm as the music commanded and when I opened my eyes they fell upon one of the coolest motherfuckers to ever set foot in this place or any other.

He was a soulful, slim cat. A young brother with boyish good looks and an easy manner about him as if every move, every glance around the room, the casual nod of his head as he dug the raw sound, were all done with an artistic economy of motion. He looked like a transplant from the late thirties, like Robert Johnson's running buddy, like a real delta bluesman traveled up the great Mississippi to Chicago. Grey suit slacks and a grey button down vest hugged his slender frame rather dashingly, and a black derby hat, slightly cocked to one side, sat faithfully perched atop his head. He had a natural way about him that was real smooth and confident, and left the impression that he had nothing to prove, ever.

The music stirred him to move and he quietly stepped to the dance floor, gracefully bobbing his shoulders, swaying his hips, tapping his feet and snapping his fingers. All of it with a beautiful, fluid ease, as if the vibrations had his limbs on tender, sensitive strings. He was real humble and smooth. You got the sense you were watching an improvisational art form as well as hearing one from the stage. The loveliest, most ravishing girl, adorned in flattering spandex jeans and shiny black heels was drawn to him, approaching him and asking for his hand. They danced with such striking fluidity that the whole floor cleared and we all watched in awe.

By the next set, the cool cat had a line of beautiful women waiting to dance with him. It never got to his head. He humbly accepted each of them as they ran up, one after the other, and twirled them around, showing them the smoothness of cool. They loved him for it because he was better than wanting anything other than a simple dance. He never desecrated the moment by drawing them too close or cheaply rubbing up against them. He always kept them at a friendly distance, making them all blush, quite by accident, with his tender smile and haunting eyes. He was quite a character and it seemed everyone appreciated him except for the dates of his dancing partners who quietly stewed until their women returned, then flashed phony smiles as if nothing was bothering them.

Costa left as last call approached for the rest of Chicago outside the glowing, woodshed walls of the Kingston Mines. "I'm done," he confessed. I listened without removing my eyes from the stage, I couldn't. "Besides, I wanna check out all the mamasitas on the sidewalk scene for last call, you know the way back, right?"

"Yeah, yeah," I said, snapping out of it to say goodbye. "Good stuff, huh?"

"Oh yeah, and I'm glad you love it, but I'm beat." I was quite oppositely charged and began eyeing the clock with a sense of dread, knowing full well that the curtain would fall at four.

The mad, divine night continued with an hourly scramble between rooms, rushing like a levee break, with the fresh and rested band picking up right before everyone made it into their room. The now "on break" band would saunter in and grab a drink at the bar, listening to their contemporaries and accepting the praises of patrons who insisted on buying them a drink. By two-thirty, a surge of new life overwhelmed the place as hoards of kids swarmed in from the casualties of last call. The young drunks seemed oddly out of place in trendy, stylish threads, and were solely there because the Kingston Mines could serve an hour past last call. The bar hoppers were drunk enough that they were swept up in the mad give and take occurring between audience and musician and filled the dance floor with a writhing mass, enjoying themselves immensely.

Almost unnoticed, a large, lumbering black man, in a black pin striped suit and a matching hat gently weaved his way through the crowd. He carried a long rectangular case and slowly made his way to a chair near the front, but to the side, slouching heavily as he sat. I thought his hulking shoulders might tear right through his suit jacket. The case rested on his great knees and he opened it carefully, like a treasure chest, revealing a beautiful, gleaming, white guitar. He intrigued a petite brunette, freckled and girlish, who could have been out to celebrate her 21st for how young she looked. Being wasted, she ambled right up and let forth a flurry of bubbly questions. He was enamored, smiling warmly at her. He almost seemed entertained by her perky, innocent interest. His giant, mitt of a hand swallowed her dainty hand to the wrist when they formally introduced themselves. It was one of those moments, like our lunch in Seattle, where strangers are the way they're supposed to be with each other.

He sat there, through the first half of the set, long after the girl ran back to her friends at the bar, and waited patiently. Occasionally he peered into his case, fingering his instrument, as if to make sure it hadn't run off too. I wanted them to let him play, and began to grow concerned he wouldn't get his chance. Finally, the burly bassist announced, "we wanna have our friend Floyd come up here and play a couple of songs with us," to which he grinned boyishly, plodding up to the stage with a sleepy, lazy gait and plugged his guitar into an amp. His large head shot outwards from his slouching, massive shoulders and his face drooped calmly and his lips fell into a pout as he focused on his solos. The rest of the time he smiled wonderfully, lighting up the stage. "Yeah Floyd," I screamed from within the crowd. I loved him.

Floyd's guitar sang like a bird. He was pious, almost monk like in his reserved manner on stage. This great mountain of a man, and his giant, thick fingers that moved like a breeze with agile purpose across the neck of his instrument, sang his six string siren so eloquently that I could feel his fingers, and the vibrating strings through his fingers, inside my chest. I can't explain how. It was wild and makes me smile to this day when I think about it. His solos were gripping, fluttering ballads, grounded poignantly in a simmering delta stew. They were tender and sturdy and unyieldingly soaked in the substance of life, like a brilliant sparrow singing faithfully through a thunderstorm. I'm talking about it too much and ruining it. He was simple and true, and I pushed my way up to the front of the sweltering crowd and peered up at him, catching it all.

The time for the last set had arrived, and the crowd herded back into the room with the old man, but he wasn't up there with this band. In his place stood this somewhat chunky brother with sparkling, square, gold rimmed glasses, a tight orange shirt and a cool light brown derby hat with a tiny orange feather sticking out of it. He looked like Bo Diddley's cousin and was a true madman, a man on fire who played at one insane, raw level of intensity the entire time he was on stage. There were no slow and steady build-ups to his solos. They were all one long, sustained explosion of furious fury, of love and hate and the eternal roar of man, howling and wailing for the pure and easy joy of it.

I felt as if my chest would burst open. "Yeeeaaahh," I screamed over and over again in the most soulful, bellowing yells. I didn't know where they came from. I was possessed. I went right up to him, teetering on my heels to the ruckus rhythm of his blues as rolling clouds of sonic fire came not just from his guitar, but from all of him, from his gaping, moaning mouth--gold tooth flashing--from his flaming soul that pulsed with such power that it arched his back and pointed itself straight to the heavens. I studied every wonderful, mean grimace that ran up his spine and contorted his face. And he played and he played and he played until my soul was an inferno and I thought smoke would start to billow from my ears and nostrils. He looked over at me and I screamed and he played harder. People were dancing behind me, but they meant nothing, not in the face of the holy cry.

I became drunk from the sound and suddenly turned to the dance floor and grabbed the tallest, sexiest girl out there by the hand and danced with her. Sober seven years and drunk out of my mind. At first I had gentlemanly aspirations, inspired by the birth of cool cat, but all these quickly fizzled away as I lost restraint and began writhing against her like an animal, grabbing her hips and thighs like she were mine. She blushed and I backed off, but not enough. She ran back to her group of friends, and I think her boyfriend, or suitor, who was glaring at me from the bar.

And the madman played on, wailing incandescently, his beefy face moaning with astonishing passion as the room flickered and flashed and smoldered into nothing more than the raw and unyielding sound, the burning from within, the blues.

But what burns? I've heard it said before that those who don't express their emotions store them in their muscles, joints, bones, and hearts, and they fester in them like a plague, wreaking havoc on their bodies and holding their spirits captive under a bitter, drab, blanket of malcontent. As I watched this wild bluesman with the gold rimmed glasses and his crazy eyes, possessed and gleaming, seemingly focused on another, timeless plane, I wondered if the greatest gift of the blues, the greatest strength, is a holy purging of all your hurt. I could almost see all his longings, all his pains, charging out of him, shooting out in the vessel of sound and exploding like a hailstorm of fireworks in the midnight sky, and all that is unbearably good about the human spirit showered down on us.

By expressing his pain, the bluesman observes his pain. And by observing his pain he realizes that he is not this pain, real as it may be, but the witness of the pain. Taoist philosopher Chung Yung says "Before sorrow, anger/longing, or fear have arisen/, you are in the center./ When these emotions appear/and you know how to see them,/ you are in harmony." A bluesman, or a blues listener, knows how to see his emotions. He can identify with the hardships of life, but by acknowledging these hardships, by openly singing about them instead of tucking the hurt away, the bluesman discovers a sense of detachment from his pain because he realizes that he is not the pain, but the observer of the pain, singing with truth from the center.

Perhaps the blues is a bonfire of all your pain and it creates the most beautiful sounds as it crackles and fumes away. These bluesmen become preachers of this holy sound, throwing matches at the kindling—the sadness, frustrations and longings—of those who feel it like they do, of those who are moved to greater heights by the sincerity of the music. And when you truly hear this majestic cry your stride is blessed by a lightness, a spring from within, your soul sprouts wings of angels and you are immersed in the moment and know that it exists and is beautiful and all encompassing.

The doors closed a little after four. I floated back to the motel in an energetic trance as some eternal note continued to wail in my head. I should have been exhausted. I should have been craving sleep, but I wasn't. I just sat in the darkness of our room and listened to the ghostly echoes of the show with a stupid grin on my face. It took me an hour to fall asleep and in another three we were up and ready to embark on the last leg of our journey across the great arching, sweltering continent, falling back in DC 4,500 miles after we set forth from Freemont California, and in only nine days. I felt great, as if I'd slept for weeks. There was a boyish energy infused in me. The little sleep I did catch had been a constant stream of the night's sounds and images and for the second time that week I felt blessed to have lived a string of wonderful moments twice.

I rode the manic energy inside me for the next eleven hours, finally surrendering to fatigue in Frederick, Maryland, right near the site I blew a flat the previous year returning from Colorado. From there Costa took the wheel. Outside Chicago we'd gotten lost in the country hills of Michigan for an hour or so and that was my last taste of the open road poetry that America spontaneously recites. Darkness descended and Midwest turned to East, and finally to Home. I'd only been gone three months, but it felt like a lifetime and I couldn't wait to pack up and go feast again. American Bread.

Unattached Action

I've never had a spiritual teacher. I've never had someone to illuminate the path for me. All I've had are a handful of books and a whole lot of pain. After 14 years I'm not sure where all this pain has gotten me. At times the physical hurt purified me in the sense that it simplified my life, stripped me of my meandering dreams of the future, slammed me down into the present and demanded that I find a way to cope with the here and now. Sometimes I stood up to the challenge and other times I buckled and failed. When I failed I resorted to self-pity or misery, when I succeeded I found a way to come to peace with the sensations of extreme physical discomfort and pain, and thus found a way to alleviate the suffering within my mind, if not my body.

Of course I know that there are many people who experience levels of pain that make my ordeal feel like a vacation and my heart goes out to them as I wonder where they find the strength to persevere. Is there some lesson in all this pain for all of us, for all the chronically ill? Does suffering cease when we accept the reality of *what is*, when we come to grips with the limitations of our bodies and cease to search for a cure? Is the need to be healthy a common sense practicality that every human has the right to strive for or a distracting luxury that undermines the liberating peace of acceptance? I struggled with these questions for nearly two years until I stumbled upon the compromise detailed earlier. The more I put that compromise into practice the more right it felt for me.

I began to analyze the compromise and realized that the Taoist concept of unattached action was the key component. Unattached action is acting purely out of the inherent virtue of an action, without being influenced by any possible results, either positive or negative. One who moves with unattached action is motivated by the natural beauty and goodness of an action, not the end rewards. It's about being engrossed in the process, not the product, enjoying the journey, instead of being preoccupied with the destination. In the *Tao Te Ching* Lao Tzu says, "With unattached action, there is nothing one cannot do." I believe he is suggesting that by narrowing our focus to the present, by observing the process instead of obsessing over the outcome, we honor the inherent virtue of our aim and give nature, the spirit, the Tao, or whatever you want to call IT, the best chance of flowing through us and aiding us in our achievement. In my case that aim is healing my body of Lyme disease.

The artist follows the path of his vision because the journey of creation is engrossing, captivating and liberating. His mind is always in the present. He doesn't act based on how he thinks his work will be received, for if he does he will have lost the natural worth of his action by anchoring himself to a certain chain of results. This kind of mindset is my inspiration when navigating my quest for health, which in a sense has become my art form. The process of healing my body, or striving to heal my body, on its own is a virtuous act. Reaching for health does not mean that I am rejecting my reality of illness in the present moment, or even reacting to my symptoms with aversion. To do so would be to act with an attachment to attaining health, but my aim is unattached action. Therefore I can commit all the energy and discipline to strive for health without becoming jaded or frustrated by a lack of progress, because progress is a result and all my actions are not attached to results, my actions of striving for health are done in and for themselves, like a musician who plays an instrument because the act draws her into the moment.

The Book of Chuang Tzu has a story of a master woodworker who carves a bell stand so beautiful that all who see it are astonished. When asked how his art achieves such beauty the woodworker responds, "Whenever I begin to carve a bell stand, I concentrate my mind. After three days of meditating, I no longer have any thoughts of praise or blame. After five days, I no longer have any thoughts of success or failure. After seven days, I'm not identified with a body. All my power is focused on my task; there are no distractions. At that point I enter the mountain forest. I examine the trees until exactly the right one appears." The fact that this wood worker has a goal to create a bell stand does not mean that he has set himself up to suffer by succumbing to a desire, by rejecting reality or *what is*. Quite the opposite. He has engrossed himself in the moment of *what is*. The suffering would come from attaching himself to praise or blame, success or failure. But, these are the end results, not the process, and the master wood worker knows that by being immersed in the art form, these results cease to exist.

To this day, I expend a great deal of energy taking care of my body. I eat all the right foods, abstain from drugs and alcohol, restrain my physical activity, and diligently maintain a varied schedule of medications; all with the goal of helping my body heal itself. From a purely mental standpoint I constantly attend to my thoughts, continuously churning out the belief that I will be healthy and releasing that belief into the universe, even when my symptoms are exacerbated, because I believe that our thoughts have some effect on reality.

In some ways I've come full circle from the days of my two-month experiment. Eleven years ago faith that I would be healthy allowed me to transcend the frustration that attachment to results can breed. By 2008 I began to question whether faith was, in and of itself, an attachment that led to suffering. Today, by undergoing a deeper examination of my thoughts, I have embraced the notion of unattached action and come to fully understand what I caught a glimpse of during the two-month experiment: there is no greater joy than the joy of the present.

The difference between faith and unattached action is a subtle shift of consciousness, a change of view. The process of trying to be healthy is an art form, and being engrossed in an art form can lead to unification with God, or the Spirit, or whatever you want to call IT. So I guess one could say that I am grateful for the opportunity to study the art of attaining health. Yesterday my neck hurt. I felt like my muscles back there were just a set of rusty cables that throbbed with each movement. I didn't get discouraged, frustrated or disheartened. This was another chance to practice my art form. I focused on my breath and immersed myself in the present. I accepted all that the moment had to offer, all the pain and discomfort, without any aversion. I observed those unpleasant sensations as I observed all the occurrences around my body, within my body, and within my mind. But at the same time I actively told myself, my body, the universe, that I would be healthy. I asked the Spirit to heal me. I did these things with a purpose and an aim. If I had focused on the product instead of the process, thus giving frustration and sadness an entrance into my mind, I would have lost the fundamental value of my actions because I would have fallen prey to the results. I try to be healthy because trying to be healthy is a beautiful thing, not because I need to be healthy. The inherent virtue of the unattached action is enough.

The funny thing is that a road trip demands unattached action as well. You can't go on the road with an itinerary of things to see or accomplish. You can have a loose plan at best. To truly enjoy the road you must be free to get lost because you never know what you may find. In order to truly absorb the experience you must purge yourself of expectations and desired results and immerse yourself in the journey rather than the destination. Again the idea of process over product arises, as well as the importance of connecting with the inherent virtue of an action, in this case a road trip, which for me is simply to move and to be moved.

As I said, anything can happen on the road. You can take one wrong turn in the night and end up 300 miles from where you thought you were heading with no other option than to keep going and see what you find, and often, if your mind is open, you'll discover that treasures await you in the most unexpected places. You may run across the perfect campsite along the side of an abandoned highway or drive for hours into the beaten night past an endless string of "no vacancy" signs until exhaustion starts to warp your thoughts like a crazy person's. You can blow a tire at the tail end of a 15-hour drive and be forced to change it as trucks roar by and all you can think of is the sweet caress of a bed. Or you may blow a radiator in the middle of the New Mexico desert, only to idle past a mechanic just when it seemed that your car would overheat and all would be lost. You may have your car stolen and you may even get it back. You may stumble across a madman who scares everyone around him shitless, but also inspires a great freedom in you. But, the only way to act around someone like that is with no expectations, because no one will teach you that anything is possible faster than a madman on a mad night.

These are only a tiny fraction of the nearly infinite moments that can spontaneously arise on the road, but they can only do so if you honor the inherent virtue of a road trip above all else: to move and to be moved. Taoist author Derek Lin says, "The Tao acts in a Wu Wei (unattached action) manner and effortlessly achieves the miracle of life. We find great inspiration in this and see the possibility to act without attachments and achieve great works without friction or resistance." On the road the greatest friction that can arise is within your mind. If you can greet each perceived obstacle with equanimity you will see that most obstacles are just different paths, all of which allow you to move and be moved.